Voices United: Collective Excellence in Autism

Nicola Myers Gardere M.ED/CI

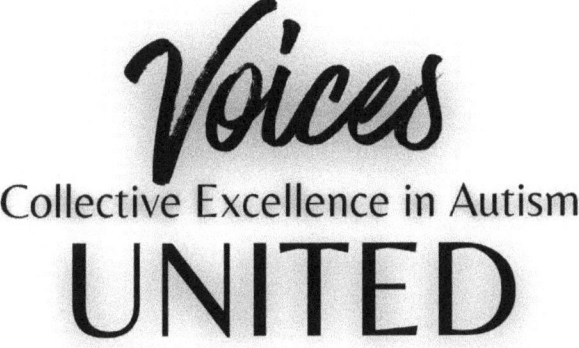

Collective Excellence in Autism

A compilation of genuine stories and personal experiences on parenting and caring for a child with autism

Voices United: Collective Excellence in Autism

This page left blank intentionally.

BLACKSEEDSPUBLISHING.
PLANTING SEEDS OF LOVE, FORGIVENESS & HEALING

Voices United: Collective Excellence in Autism

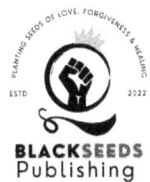

Copyright © 2023 by Nicola Myers Gardere

All rights reserved. No part of this publication may be reproduced, distributed, or transmitted in any form or by any means, including photocopying, recording, or other electronic or mechanical methods, without the prior written permission of the publisher, except in the case of brief quotations embodied in critical reviews and certain other noncommercial uses permitted by copyright law. For permission requests, write to the publisher at the address below.

Black Seeds Publishing
support@blackseedspublishing.com
www.blackseedspublishing.com

The views expressed in this publication are those of the author and do not necessarily reflect the official policy or position of any other agency, organization, employer or company associated with the publisher.

Scripture quotations taken from the Holy Bible, King James Version, unless otherwise noted.

Printed in the United States of America

ISBN-13: 979-8-9878956-8-9

I would like to dedicate this book to families across the globe working with autustic children. Continue to prioritize their needs and you will see excellence in everything they touch. -Nicola

> When a flower doesn't bloom you fix the environment in which it grows, not the flower.
> –Alexander Den Heijer

This page left blank intentionally.

BLACKSEEDSPUBLISHING.
PLANTING SEEDS OF LOVE, FORGIVENESS & HEALING

Table of Contents

About the Book Collaboration..9

Chapter 1
Excellence in Autism by Nicola Gardere 13

Chapter 2
Raising Jiraiya by Melesia Hudson.............................44

Chapter 3
The Neurodi-Way by msMISSYms 94

Chapter 4
Autism From an Outside Perspective by Evelyn Prewitt 125

Conclusion 135

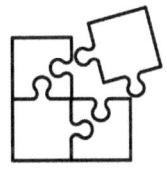

Voices United: Collective Excellence in Autism

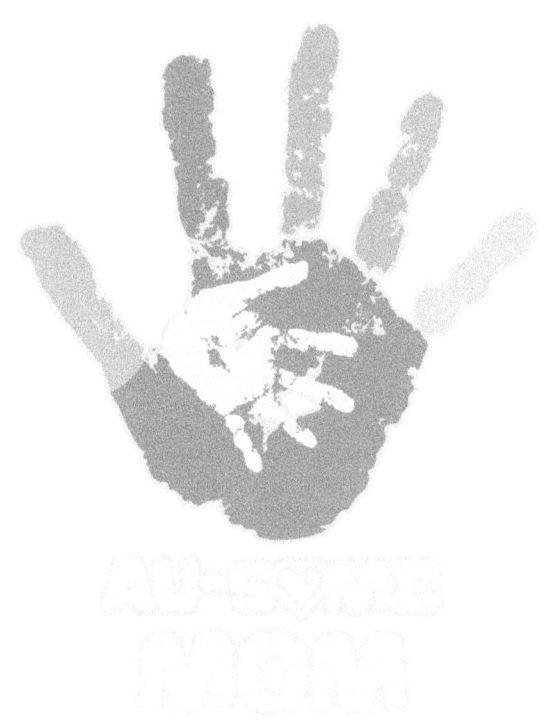

About the Book Collaboration

Education is my lifelong passion and the individuals I have met over the last 20 years create a space for me to evolve into the best version of myself while changing lives. Amazingly, all the women in this collaboration I met though my interactions working with children, after the first two minutes of meeting, our voices became a collective sound and we decided to march to the same beat.

Most people know that when life gets the best of me, exercise is my escape to refocus and realign. Many years ago while engaging in my 5am exercise routines, I met the beautiful Melissa, with a heart for changing lives and helping others find their inner strengths. Melissa pushed my fitness levels to the maximum to a point of running the 450 steps stadium bleacher has become my ultimate favorite way to release and challenge myself.

I soon realized that her passion and strength was unmatchable, being able to coach individuals beyond what they felt they could master is an art. Upon learning that she parented a child with autism, it was easy for me to invite her to the team to share her strength of parenting and resilience to help others.

Missy, Missy as I love to chant her name, we met several years ago on a service project though our university on the beautiful island of Jamaica. Not only did I find value in her friendship, but it was also a sight to behold when the country immediately embraced her warmth and her love for people.

Being her roommate for 10 days on 7 miles of beautiful white sandy beaches in Negril we bonded over success stories she shared on her techniques of working with children and adults. Listening to the smash ups and brain hacks that she provides for all children and especially the autistic community made this collaborative decision easy.

Evelyn and I met on a middle school campus working with children. Her passion and dedication will leave you thanking God for the gift he placed in her to help others. As an educator and case worker she goes above and beyond to ensure all children are treated fairly and experience the joy of inclusion.

On any given day her faith precedes her in her conversation and actions. Inviting her to the team was an easy decision because her heart lies in serving others.

Serving as the visionary author on this project fills me with gratitude that others felt compelled to join this collaboration. We stand as voices united for children.

-Nicola

"

Be still, and know that I am God: I
will be exalted among the heathen, I
will be exalted in the earth.
-Psalm 46:10

Chapter 1

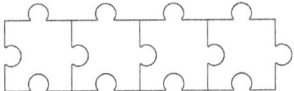

Excellence In Autism By Nicola Gardere

As the years slowly ticked by, I was acutely aware that something was *different*. The sounds, movements, and responses were different, and I was amazed at the richness of the life we were blessed with.

We soon realized we were in the presence of excellence and talent beyond words. The kids were inquisitive and asked many questions.

Why the constant movements, why the outburst, why did unusual look so normal to us but different to others? I promised we would discover together and embrace the excellence that existed in our own backyard.

As a Program Director serving multiple facilities, I traveled all over the region, providing training and support to administrators and support staff, not knowing that I would be forever connected to this level of excellence and talent through one person. The challenge for me showed up when I had to spend some time completing an investigation at the Children's Center in Austin.

One Friday evening, after spending the day at the children's center, I recall crying out and asking why the children seemed so unaware of what lay ahead in society for them. The level of innocence and trust that they had within them fueled something inside of me to fight for others to see the excellence that they were, at times, unable to articulate.

With social skills lacking in many, it became apparent that my work to bring awareness just began. And, oh yes, I became their biggest cheerleader!

My work soon spoke for itself, and I was asked to attend training as a facilities investigator for the company. My role in this capacity allowed me to work closely with staff and clients to ensure they had the best representation and a voice that would never be silenced.

And it is this work that has lead me to write this book to share, not only my story, but others who have witnessed and experienced the same—living with or caring for a child with a autism.

What is autism, some may ask? As an educator and a parent, understanding autism was puzzling for me. Questions that plagued my mind surrounded equity, quality of life, safety, and security.

Webster's dictionary defines autism as:

> A variable developmental disorder that appears by age three and is characterized especially by difficulties in forming and maintaining social relationships, by impairment of the ability to communicate verbally or nonverbally, and by repetitive behavior patterns restricted interests and activities.

Research shows **Autism Spectrum Disorder** is the term most frequently used to describe deficits in social communication, repetitive behaviors, and several other causes. With more inclusive practices and training, children diagnosed with autism have a brighter future ahead than other children had over 50 years ago (Elsabbagh, Baird & Veenstra-Vanderweele, 2018).

What did this all mean, and what was I walking into as a parent and an educator with several children depending on me to be successful, both socially and academically? I needed help figuring out where to start.

I began indulging in the research while teaching my children how to be patient with their baby brother. While my older son was more tolerant of the behaviors, my younger son had no idea what to do or how to manage the difference that he saw, which later manifested itself into excellence. The kids soon found out they had more similarities than differences.

Investigating cases from exploitation to abuse showed me how vulnerable our children were and how unkind society can sometimes be.

Carry the Glory of God Wherever You Go!

Growing up in a family with a preaching grandmother, we often heard this phrase spoken boldly. Grandma often reminds us of God's words to suffer the little children to come unto me and forbid them not.

Chapter 1: Excellence in Autism

> Jesus said, "Let the little children come to me, and do not hinder them, for the kingdom of heaven belongs to such as these."
> -Matthew 19:14 (NIV)

I now know that regardless of what behavior challenges and embarrassment one may encounter because of what different looks like, we must press on and ensure that the right supports are in place to support families of children who behave differently and have different cognitive challenges. Manifesting this behavior through kindness, respect, and humility will ensure we treat others equally.

❦

My first teaching assignment was in a psychiatric hospital in Texas. I was quickly exposed to various levels of disability. Most prevalent in the hospital were children with emotional challenges. However, I was quickly introduced to a 4th grader, whom I will call Seth.

After being around Seth for less than an hour, I started seeing the differences in his behaviors. However, I realized that he was more *like* the other kids on my attendance roster, than he was *different* from them.

The lesson planning looked different because I had to ensure Seth had access to what he was entitled to. Explaining to the children that one may need more support to access the same thing will help them understand that this was the best approach to delivering equitable practices; they deserved the explanation but not the intrusion into other students' cases.

I loved Sundays when I would sit around to review Seth's progress and/or regress and use that data to plan for him. One of my mentors often reminded us to "make the main thing the main thing." All my students were the main ones. Still, Seth required more deliberate planning to ensure the playing field was level.

I recall sitting in one of Seth's treatment teams, providing updates and solutions that we believed would help him succeed. I turned to him and asked him what he needed from us. He shyly looked away and said, "I just want to be treated like the other kids by everyone and not just you."

That hit the spot for me and set off a wave of advocacy I had never felt before. What if all kids felt this way but did not know how to verbalize or communicate it? Knowing that we have autistic students who are verbal and nonverbal required me to start fighting for them all.

Something quite fascinating that I noticed in my interactions with children with autism. Along with the stimming, I have also experienced the fixation on topics of interest. *If this is the first time you have observed or noticed this, keep an eye out.*

What is *stimming*? Webster's Dictionary defines it as:

> A self-stimulatory behavior marked by repetitive action or movement of the body and typically associated with certain conditions such as Autism spectrum disorder.

Seth had a deep fixation on technology; he would sit and talk about any electronic devices he saw fit. He was very knowledgeable and spent a great deal of time watching videos and asking questions.

It was an interesting combination--while his word recognition was on the high school level, his comprehension level was that of an elementary student. Working with Seth opened many doors that I experienced in my childhood years.

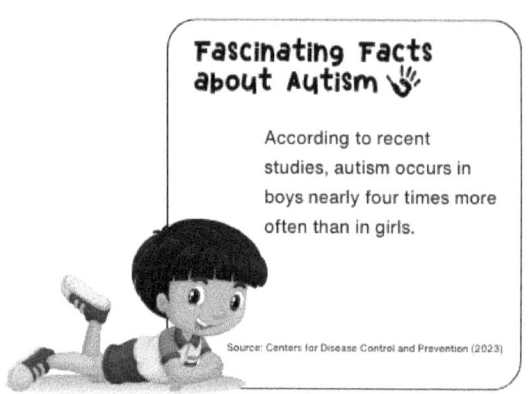

Fascinating Facts about Autism

According to recent studies, autism occurs in boys nearly four times more often than in girls.

Source: Centers for Disease Control and Prevention (2023)

Growing up on the beautiful island of Jamaica in my younger years, our daily lives were routine. I enjoyed the banana or cornmeal porridge you could smell coming from the kitchen every morning or the smell of fresh peppermint tea, attending to my chores and getting dressed for school.

I loved my childhood; I recall being kind to everyone. I may not have made physical contact because we were told the behaviors of the special population were, at times, impulsive, so we kept our distance.

The interesting fact is that they did not bother us; I might even think they protected us because we were familiar faces. However, the life of an adult or child with a disability looks different through our eyes. As the memories began to crash in, I wondered how many children and/or adults felt this way that I encountered.

Growing up as a little girl, I recall visiting my maternal grandmother every summer, and some long weekends. There was one young lady, I will call her Emma, who had a fixation on me for some reason; she had a name she affectionately called me, which was Chaaaattola... I assumed that is how it sounded due to her speech impediment.

I, on the other hand, was terrified of this lady. I dreaded passing her home and would muster up all my energy to run as fast as I could before she saw me and attempted to come near. Oh, how I feared the unknown of what looked *different* to me as a child.

With no explanations, I feared her sound; I feared the approaches; I feared different because different, without explanations, can be frightening.

I now look back at those days and wish someone had taken the time to explain to me why she behaved differently. Maybe they didn't know, or we would have heard the private conversations of the adults we sometimes walked into before being told to stay in a child's place, which meant to go back and play with our siblings or peers and not enter the conversations of the grown-ups.

A typical day for Miss Emma was spent sitting on the side of her family home. She hummed and stimmed, whether that was moving back and forth or fast hand movements that were repetitive and constant.

One thing was evident with Miss Emma, and it was the fact that she was well-cared for by her family. While they were always close by, I do not recall seeing any communication that would lead me to believe that deliberate steps were taken to grow her in other areas outside of daily living skills.

How much did she understand, or were most of her responses based on learned behaviors? I recall one-word commands being given: *Come, Dinner.*

As I write, my childhood memories overwhelm me because I wish I could go back with this knowledge and expertise to make a difference. I don't recall Grandma stating that Miss Emma went to public or trade school because, in the 1960s, the Island needed programs focused on those areas.

How much potential was locked inside her, and what behaviors could have been learned to change her quality of life? One will never know, or at least I will never know.

Chapter 1: Excellence in Autism

While I was in middle school, I recall visiting my Grandma, and for the first time, I did not run past Miss Emma's home or fear going by because Grandma shared that she was gravely ill.

I felt a wave wash over me; regardless of the fear I grappled with, Miss Emma became a part of my visits to Grandma's. Not seeing her felt different.

I asked Grandma if I could visit with her one evening. See, back in the day, when someone was dying, close community and family members sat in the room as they transitioned. I asked Grandma if I could sit in the room with the elders as they hummed or sang.

I was in the same room for the first time and did not have to run. She looked so peaceful and calm as she lay there. I remember feeling an overwhelming sadness; why did I allow her stillness and calm to give me a sense of protection?

As she took her last breath, my Grandma took me out of the room. I trembled and silently waved goodbye, knowing I would never see her alive again. I wonder how often Miss Emma wanted me to be still and accept her for being her. Nothing about her seemed *different* to her because that girl--that body--was all she knew.

How often do we run from things or situations that may help us grow, but allow the unknown to trap us into thinking *different* is just too different?

Years later, as an adult visiting my home island again, I recently passed by Miss Emma's home while attending my Aunt Pearl's funeral. I looked towards the area where she often stood and the silence was deafening, I longed to hear her call my name one more time.

I wanted to tell her that *I hear you* and *I see you*. I wanted her to know that I no longer must run from her because we were more alike than we were different. I wonder what she would have done had I gone to her after her beckon. Would she touch my face, hold my hand, or grab me due to a lack of impulse control?

All these unanswered questions raced through my mind. Unfortunately, I will never know. I allowed the fear of the unknown to rob me of that experience. I now know better as an educator, and I plan to share the knowledge I have gained over the years to change lives.

BEING THE VOICE FOR YOUR CHILD: TIPS FOR PARENTS

Parenting a child with autism is both rewarding and challenging. Due to the child's difficulties with expressive language and social skills, parenting involves considering various aspects such as education, society, health, and even financial responsibilities.

To be an effective parent requires being involved in all aspects of their lives. Knowing how your child learns best will give you the knowledge you need to advocate for them. Many parents with autistic children are learning alongside them.

Being proactive and sharing information with teachers, therapists, and anyone involved in their children's lives will only increase your knowledge and provide the best support system for your child.

Being intentional about the experiences and environment we create for our children is critical. Setting up a system that will change their mindsets will create habits that will benefit them throughout life.

Our children should know that they matter and they deserve the best. Parents must be committed to the journey of encouraging and raising productive citizens regardless of disabilities.

As an educator, parent of two young men, and sibling to someone who requires specialized services, we often find ourselves grappling with questions, experiencing sleepless nights, and constantly learning about new topics.

Research shows that when a child with autism enters the world, the family will experience changes in the family dynamics, which sometimes is seen as a natural crisis period.

Parenting a child with autism has many complexities that create additional family stressors, starting with communication. No communication manual is handed to each parent once their child has been diagnosed with autism.

Webster's dictionary defines communication as:

> The exchange of thoughts, opinions or information by speech, writing or nonverbal expression. Language is communication using words--written, spoken or signed.

Chapter 1: Excellence in Autism

Here's a hard core truth: Children with autism communicate differently than the typically developing child. And that's okay.

Working in a special education environment, I noticed that the nonverbal and verbal cues from the children were not always met with a favorable response by the staff. However, one must understand and be willing to sacrifice the time required to ensure all students can access the resources to create a thriving environment.

Autistic children use language differently from their non-disabled peers and often communicate through behaviors. It is typical to hear made-up words mimic or repeat words heard in their environment that may derive from their favorite TV shows, TikTok, and YouTube.

Children diagnosed with autism communicate slightly differently when using nonverbal cues. At a very young age, my son's younger brother sometimes used my hand to point to an object or the direction he wanted to go. Not getting his way within the timeframe, he sometimes shifted his gaze to his brothers.

We must be intentional and deliberate in our communication with the children. Working with autistic children in communication must occur in multiple steps. I encourage parents to observe the behaviors displayed by the children and plan strategically how they will improve communication and when to introduce new steps.

Visual representations will help the child make connections. Allow them to hear one instruction at a time and allow them to complete or attempt such a task. Once a skill is mastered, it becomes harder to unlearn because most things are taken literally.

I often apply to the Gradual Release of Responsibility (GRR) process. As an educator, we often associate GRR as stages through a lesson cycle. However, I believe in consistency and being deliberate. Using some of the techniques at home that are seen in the classroom will only enhance that skill and ensure the exposure is consistent.

I often model the task for students with autism, then we do it together, and as a proud supporter or cheerleader, I step back and watch them execute.

Patience and consistency must exist in the same space for the autistic child to be successful; it will take an autistic child longer to process and retain information.

Chapter 1: Excellence in Autism

Knowing that children with autism require special space will help us create a safe and calm environment for them. Sensory overloads create anxiety and chaos for children.

A classroom with 15 children, which does not seem like a lot until you add disabilities into the equation, will expose the need for space to be prioritized.

I recall one far corner of my classroom being the reading center. I have a reading tree with several bean bags and books for the students. When behaviors escalated in the classroom, I noticed Seth would make his way to the tree and just lay there sometimes with his hands over his ears.

A contingency plan had to be implemented immediately to ensure his well-being was prioritized. Seth and I met with a buddy teacher one classroom over, and she allowed him to visit for a few minutes each day to help him become familiar with her classroom and students.

She also had a space for him to sit and read if I needed additional support. Soon, this became our safety net. Seth knew if the behaviors escalated in my classroom, grabbing his pass and going next door would help him manage the stressors around him.

One may think this is easier done at school because we can send the student to a buddy teacher that they are familiar with. Creating a space at home may be as simple as going into the den or the parent's room to relax or calm down.

My stepson often found peace and a secure space in my bedroom. With a recliner in one area, that was his spot if he needed to calm down or unwind from feelings of anxiety. Keeping in mind self-regulation of behaviors will reduce anxiety for both you and the child who is experiencing the stress.

Parents and educators must have systems for predictable patterns to help them transition. Consistency is the key to ensuring that the autistic child is comfortable and that we are creating the best environment for them to thrive.

As parents, we have several irons in the fire, as my mom Elaine would often say. However, prioritizing the time it takes to communicate and offering positive praise and/or rewards will only help to reinforce and strengthen the capacity of the child to move to the next level of communication.

Chapter 1: Excellence in Autism

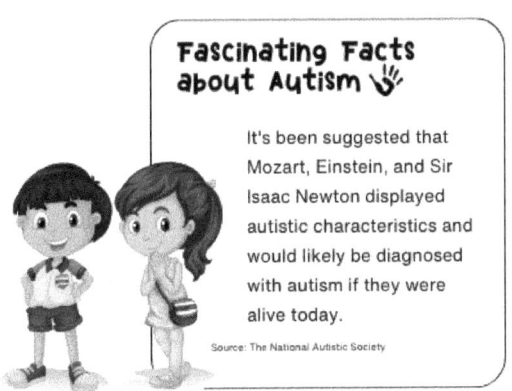

CIRCLE UP! LET'S TALK

As a trainer of restorative practices, I spend considerable time facilitating circles with students, community leaders, and parents. I have worked with autistic students for the past 17 years and realize the circle design for autistic children looks slightly different.

During my research, there is evidence to support the benefits students gain from this practice. This practice will improve behaviors and social interactions with others.

During a circle experience, the focus is on communication, and most students with autism struggle in that area. Being patient and hearing the same question helps them respond, whether orally or in pictures.

Restorative circles will help students feel safe communicating and increase their ability to participate in social settings.

Among some commonalities with what felt different was the ability to sit and listen while others were talking and not interrupting.

I was excited to return to Jamaica a few years ago, and as detailed in my best-seller book "Circle Up Let's Talk," I was excited to see the students in an inclusive setting working alongside their peers.

While inclusion looked slightly different from how it was presented in the United States, it warmed my heart to see the students interacting with their peers in one classroom and not singled out.

I was more encouraged to see several organizations providing support to families. The Autism Foundation of Jamaica is an excellent resource for parents on the island looking for answers or solutions to care for their special needs child. While on the island, I hosted several training sessions with teachers and students in Negril.

At first, the students felt awkward with this way of communicating because it was *different*. During the restorative circles, one of the essential components required everyone in the circle to listen while others were speaking.

I would now like to share with you what the *circle process* looks like in Chapter 7 of *Circle Up, Let's Talk*:

> For lasting change to occur, it must occur across all environments. I firmly believe in what my Grandma Miranda preached for years: "Train up a child in the way he should go and when he gets old, he will not depart from it." - Proverbs 22:6, KJV
>
> This rings true especially for me as an administrator, working with students from various backgrounds and socio-economic status, enforcing expectation is a challenging process because everyone parents differently and sees occurrences through different lenses.

Parents nationwide can benefit from restorative parenting training on how to communicate with children rather than imposing punitive consequences. Teaching the children at home how to communicate with each other will create an atmosphere of trust and respect both at home and radiate through the hallways of every campus.

It is impossible to tell any parent how to parent. However, I firmly believe it takes a village to raise a child, and we must work together to ensure all our children are well. While parents have a responsibility to care for their children, we must never neglect the art of teaching them how to love and respect others.

What does restorative parenting look like? Working with students in an age where they have so much access to the world wide web, we must be cognizant of the fact they are being exposed to things we are not aware of. Sitting with our children is more critical now than ever.

Relationships take time, and children must listen to themselves and others. I cannot begin to tell you how many times I cringe in my seat when I hear parents say, "you won't amount to anything," "I can't stand you," "You don't deserve my time." All these words are damaging, and we must find ways as parents to start repairing the harm that is being done to children.

I am certain what we teach our youth, they will carry into the future. We must find meaningful and intentional ways to break this generational behavior that has plagued our families for centuries.

CIRCLE UP IN ACTION

When working with an autistic child in a circle, you may have to adjust the norms to provide support to help the student communicate by modeling and prompting. What is important is that you clearly communicate that before the circle starts and during the process.

Circle Up looks just like a circle; all parties are either sitting on the floor, or on chairs, but must be in a circle with no barriers. Once in our new circle-up room, each student took a seat, and I went over the group norms with the class to help them understand the expectations. They were all in agreement. I asked them to add a few expectations of their own since this was our group.

After a consensus of the expectations, I then described what the centerpiece was and what it represented; the centerpiece represents the collective in the group and must be something of value.

For instance, a centerpiece for an athletic circle could be a basketball, volleyball, frisbee, uniform, etc. I am sure you will get the picture here. The talking piece was introduced next, and of course, everyone wanted to hold the item that represented the talking piece; the talking piece is an object that is of value and importance to the students.

During the circle process, only the individual holding the talking piece is talking; this increases active listening for others in the group and sends a strong message that what you have to say is equally important.

My choir teacher uses a microphone as her talking piece, whereas my band teacher may use a drumming stick, something that represents the collective and is of value.

After engaging in a value round, the kids were amazed to hear the values of each other and who taught it to them. I could tell they struggled with waiting their turn since they were not allowed to speak without the talking piece.

This can be challenging for adults like me who may need to use a talking piece to avoid interrupting others.

It may be common to go through a practice round to help the children understand the process since this may be new for most. With the same questions being asked of everyone in the circle, the children may react more favorably.

I encourage parents and educators not to give up. Hosting a Circle can be challenging, requiring patience even for those without disabilities. It may take several circles for the family to be comfortable. I promise you the reward will be far greater than the sacrifice.

Both the children and the families need support to ensure the autistic child experiences the least amount of stress in the quest to be gainfully employed and or live independent lives.

I encourage parents to get in touch with their local government offices to find out the resources that are available to their child. Educators and parents must be aware of the support and services available to help students globally.

The experiences shared in this book will help families understand how to connect and empower each other while on this challenging journey. Knowing where you are with caring for your child will help you create a roadmap for success.

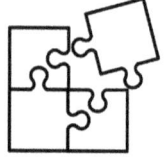

REFERENCES

Lord, C., Elsabbagh, M., Baird, G., & Veenstra-Vanderweele, J. (2018). Autism spectrum disorder. https://doi.org/10.1016/S0140-6736(18)31129-2

What does Autism stand for in medical terms? Rhumbarlv.com. https://www.rhumbarlv.com/what-does-autism-stand-for-in-medical-terms/

Identification and Evaluation of children with Autism https://publications.aap.org/pediatrics/article/120/5/1183/71081/Identification-and-Evaluation-of-Children-With

Parenting of children with autism spectrum disorder https://www.ncbi.nlm.nih.gov/pmc/articles/PMC8306821/

Autism Spectrum Disorder https://www.sciencedirect.com/science/article/abs/pii/S0140673618311292

Gardere, N. Circle up Let's Talk, Jai Publishing House, 2020

ABOUT THE AUTHOR

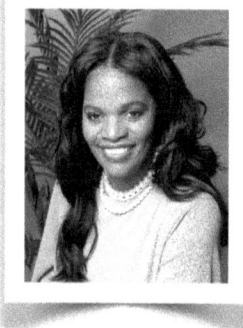

Ms. Gardere is a distinguished professional who currently serves as a High School Administrator in Texas, bringing with her a wealth of experience spanning over two decades.

Her dedication lies in the realm of education, with a particular focus on catering to special populations, ranging from elementary to post-secondary levels.

In her impressive career, Ms. Gardere has held the position of Vocational Rehabilitation Director in the Central Texas area and El Paso, where she skillfully managed the vocational rehabilitation department for a private assisted living company. Her work primarily revolved around providing vital services to both adults and children with special needs.

Beyond her administrative roles, Ms. Gardere has carved a notable niche as an accomplished author, with two Amazon best-selling books to her name: "Live your Abundant Life Too" and "Circle Up! Let's Talk (Restorative Discipline Practices for Educators)."

Additionally, she has authored the "Moving Forward Journal," available in both Spanish and English. Her literary contributions have made a significant impact, offering valuable insights to a diverse readership.

Notably, Ms. Gardere extends her influence on a global scale as an international guest speaker, contributing her expertise and knowledge to audiences worldwide. She is not only a dedicated mother but also a Doctoral Scholar, highlighting her commitment to continuous learning and growth.

Family holds a special place in Ms. Gardere's heart, as she takes pride in being the mother of two young men and a loving grandmother to a seven-year-old granddaughter and a one-year-old grandson. Her personal experiences have equipped her with a unique perspective on understanding the challenges of spending time with a stepchild with Autism and Traumatic Brain Injury (TBI).

Ms. Gardere's passion for advocacy extends to national and international stages, where she has presented at various conferences, emphasizing the importance of serving special needs children and promoting restorative conversations to ensure that every voice is heard and validated.

She is a dedicated servant leader and an active volunteer, generously giving her time and expertise to numerous organizations, both locally and abroad. Ms. Gardere's influence extends to the legislative sphere, where she collaborates with legislators in the state of Texas through the Texas Policy Institute. Her contributions focus on amending and reviewing policies within the Public and Higher Education sector, with a vision to benefit all students.

Beyond her professional endeavors, Ms. Gardere is the CEO of the Myers Gardere International Foundation, which champions the cause of restoring communities through purposeful giving on a global scale. Her "Feed the Need" program has successfully launched events in Jamaica and Nigeria, ensuring that no family goes to bed hungry. She is also an esteemed member of Zeta Phi Beta Sorority Inc., further demonstrating her commitment to community and sisterhood.

Ms. Gardere's multifaceted contributions encompass education, literature, advocacy, and philanthropy, making her an inspiring figure with a profound impact on her community and the world.

Contact Nicola
- Nicolagardere.com
- www.myersgarderefoundation.org

"

At the end of the day, the most overwhelming key to a child's success is the positive involvement of parents.
-Jane D. Hull

Chapter 2

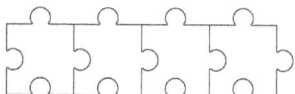

Raising Jiraiya By Melesia Hudson

I am writing this to you as a 37-year-old mother of three. My profession by day is an elementary school teacher. At this point in my life, I have a 17-year-old son, a 14-year-old daughter, and a 5-year-old son.

My 5-year-old is Jiraiya. He is the one who is diagnosed as having Autism Spectrum Disorder. In writing this, I hope to offer hope and guidance and to let you know that you are not alone.

Chapter 2: Raising Jiraiya

I didn't think anything was *different*, nor did I have a different experience with Jiraiya in the early stages of life. Pregnancy was normal. I ate the right foods and continued exercising because that was always important to me. I was admitted to the hospital at 39 weeks. I was induced because my obstetrician was going out of town, and I didn't want anyone unfamiliar delivering my baby.

I gave birth on December 20, 2016. I was happy and so in love. I delivered a beautiful baby boy that evening, and as I held him, I knew instantaneous love for the third time. I took him home the next day and introduced Jiraiya to his siblings, Mavric and Mikaila.

The weeks following delivery were blissful. I snuggled, nursed, rocked, sang, and, most of all, enjoyed every single moment I could.

The early days were ordinary. Jiraiya met his developmental milestones whenever he was expected to. He smiled at me when I talked to him. He cooed and was happy around those he loved. I would hold, nurse, and make eye contact with him. He was a happy baby with a smile that lit up my world.

When it was time to return to work, I walked in and saw one of my co-workers and broke down, saying, "I can't do this." She assured me it would be okay, but as mothers, I don't think we're ever ready to leave our babies. It goes against our nature as mothers, nurturers, and caretakers to these individuals who grew inside our bellies and with whom we share a soul.

I went to work, and during this time, a wonderful Puerto Rican lady named Myriam looked after my child as if he was her own. She would send me pictures of him sleeping or when she would comb his hair over. He had the most beautiful, curly head of hair. I would giggle and show off the pictures to anyone around me.

That summer, when Jiraiya was 7 months old, Jiraiya's dad, who we'll call Jim, was sent to Afghanistan on contract work. He left every few months, so nothing was really out of the norm. I didn't stress; I didn't feel helpless. My life was as perfect as I thought it could be. I had my babies, a beautiful home, and a promising career. All was as close to perfect as I thought it could be.

I worked as a full-time Pre-K teacher while Jiraiya stayed with his sitter during the day. My daughter attended the school where I was a teacher, and my son participated at the local middle school. Jiraiya's dad arrived around November, a few weeks before he turned one. Things were a little strained, but I didn't think anything about it. I chalked it up to the stress of being gone for months away from his family and the readjustment period.

He grew more distant, nitpicking things that never bothered him before. One night, he purchased a secondary phone, and that immediately sent me into a whirlwind of emotions—this man had a history of infidelity. I believed this phone had something to do with this.

I became enraged, threw something on the ground, and stormed off. He followed me and said he wanted a divorce if I didn't pick it up. I didn't really believe him at the time. I thought it would blow over. No, he eventually did end up filing for divorce.

A couple months later, after reviewing phone records, there were two numbers that he would call and would talk to for hours upon hours daily. I contacted one of them, and sure enough, it was his "friend." she said he was helping her with VA paperwork. They are now married. Guess that suspicion about the second phone was right after all.

We moved out that April, and I was awarded full custody. Jiraiya was about 15-months-old at this time. Jim chose to maintain the previously established schedule while we all lived together: he would work all day and then personal train in the evenings and weekends. This really limited his time with Jiraiya. Due to this, he could pick him up every other weekend beginning on Saturday at noon.

I had asked Myriam, his sitter, if she would speak Spanish to him so he could be bilingual. That was always a dream of mine and something I felt would benefit him in the future.

At this time, Jiraiya was not speaking or communicating appropriately for his age. I assumed that this language delay was caused by him hearing two different languages. I believe this created confusion, and he didn't know which words to use appropriately. I even took him to a pediatrician to discuss the language delay, which was also validated in my belief.

According to the Center for Disease Control and Prevention, some of the language or communication milestones I should notice are:

Chapter 2: Raising Jiraiya

- Tries to say one or two words besides "mama" or "dada," like "ba" for ball or "da" for dog
- Looks at a familiar object when you name it
- Follows directions given with both a gesture and words. For example, he gives you a toy when you hold your hand out and say, "Give me the toy."
- Points to ask for something or to get help

In our spare time, Jiraiya was only interested in watching the "Color Crew" and flipping through pages of books. If the Color Crew came on, his arms started flapping like crazy. I knew it was how he showed excitement. Still, honestly, I thought this was something all toddlers did if their vocabulary wasn't strong enough to express excitement. It didn't even occur to me that there was an underlying cognitive reason for this type of behavior.

I turned to Google. The first thing that popped up were articles about Autism Spectrum Disorder. I didn't really believe this for my son. I thought there had to be another cause for the arm flapping. Self-stimulation or "stimming" was not a part of my everyday vocabulary at that point.

I called ECI (Early Childhood Intervention) in the town that I lived in. I had previously contacted them for my oldest son because he was also a delayed speaker. I didn't expect much, but I thought they could point me in the right direction for the resources to help Jiraiya.

I wasn't sure how they determined eligibility, but according to the Texas Health & Human Services Commission, ECI eligibility is determined as follows:

- ☑ Your child is evaluated using a state-approved evaluation tool to determine eligibility.
- ☑ If your child qualifies for services, the team identifies your child's strengths and needs in your family's daily routines.
- ☑ Based on the evaluation and assessment results, your team develops a plan for services, also known as the Individualized Family Service Plan (IFSP).
- ☑ Under the Individuals with Disabilities Education Act (IDEA), evaluations, assessments, and IFSPs are provided at no cost to parents."

It's an excellent resource for parents and caretakers of children who are believed to have developmental delays. It's better to know and to start getting services immediately rather than wait around and waste valuable time getting the help needed for your child.

The appointment was in June 2019. Jiraiya and I walked into the office, and I began filling out a questionnaire. The evaluator, who was so sweet and patient, started asking him questions, showing him ways to stack blocks, asking for objects around him, etc.

He wasn't interested in anything she had to say or in showing her attention at all. He wanted to eat Cheerios, and that was his focus. He couldn't identify body parts, didn't point to what he wanted, and didn't respond when his name was called. These are all "red flags" in the developmental world.

I was told we would qualify for ECI services, including a specialized skill interventionist (SSI), a speech therapist, and an occupational therapist. There are other interventions as well, and the program uses a Family Cost Share to determine out-of-pocket costs.

EARLY INTERVENTION IS KEY

We began the therapy process within the next few weeks. Jiraiya had not been to a Developmental Pediatrician, but these were steps we needed to take because early intervention is essential to help children with Autism Spectrum Disorder (ASD).

A 2007 study evaluated children who were diagnosed around age 2 and received various early interventions, including speech, behavioral, occupational, and special education. By age 4, just slightly more than half the children met the diagnostic criteria for autism, and just seven out of 10 remained on the autism spectrum.

However, the same research team noted that it is not typical of what has been seen in other studies. In one study, one out of 80 children with autism at age 2 had moved higher on the ASD spectrum by age 9, and about 20 percent of those had moved out of the spectrum.

One day, it is my hope that early intervention may even erase the signs of autism altogether.

Chapter 2: Raising Jiraiya

Next, I scheduled an appointment with Jiraiya's primary care pediatrician to get a referral, or to see if they could help me get him to sleep, which at the time was non-existent. I would begin rocking him around 7:30 p.m. and rock him to sleep until 10–11 p.m.

Jiraiya was happy to be awake by 2 or 3 a.m. the following day. It seemed like he ran on a battery, and didn't need much for it to be fully charged, so he was ready to go.

During this time, there were more battles to be fought with his dad. Although his dad worked during the day and I did not due to my profession, he was upset that the therapy sessions would not be at his house.

I didn't know how to handle this because I didn't think it was a big deal, considering Jiraiya was over there only a few days out of the month. He called to request that appointments be moved immediately to his house and let them know his displeasure.

Since Jiraiya stayed with a sitter on weekdays from 7:00 a.m.-4:00 p.m., it was in his best interest that she was trained to work with him since he would spend most of the daytime there.

A few months pass, and I hear a knock at my apartment door. I am being subpoenaed by Jim, calling for a modification of custody. Jim wants Jiraiya to live with him full time and for me to have weekend visitations. The affidavit is as follows:

> "Jiraiya has displayed concerning behavior and is developmentally behind, leading my wife and I to believe that he is neglected."

I remember thinking of all the times that I stayed home with Jiraiya. I was the one who stayed with him for 15 weeks after he was born. I was the one who would call out and take off of work if he was sick or had a well-baby appointment.

It was me and him in the evenings and most weekends while his dad was at work, training at a local gym, or working out. I had spent all of the time with him, and I didn't understand why, out of nowhere, I was being asked to relinquish my time with my baby based on being an "unfit parent."

Me and his dad didn't get along anymore, not since he decided to pursue a relationship during our marriage with his VA friend, and especially not since he immediately brought the other woman at all custody exchanges.

Chapter 2: Raising Jiraiya

He had told hideous stories of me to common friends or people I knew; all I could do was smile and continue building a life for me and my kids. I didn't think it was fair for Jiraiya to be exposed to all this negativity.

At the time, we had an ad-litem familiar with family law but didn't understand autism and what was needed for Jiraiya to feel safe, loved, and consistent in his care. I think this is a huge dilemma in the family court system, but that's a different subject for another time.

She immediately started switching the schedule around, and while Jiraiya only stayed with his dad every other weekend, she then added a Thursday overnight and claimed that it's what Texas is doing now. Again, not really considering what was best for Jiraiya.

As part of our agreement, she [the ad-litem] then discussed having Jiraiya tested for autism because the appointment that I made for him had to be scheduled a year out. She also "asked" (or more told us) that me and his dad would start doing co-parenting counseling to try to mend the relationship.

In February 2020, when Jiraiya was a little over 3-years-old, he was referred to Angela Welch, a Licensed Marriage and Family Therapist (LMFT) who used the Autism Diagnostic Observation Schedule, Second Edition (ADOS-2) to make the formal diagnosis.

She noted in the patient summary about Jiraiya's communication:

> Regarding communication, Jiraiya primarily displayed single word speech that typically consisted of one word and at times only sound per utterance.

She also observed,

> Jiraiya did not display any instances of showing items to mother and examiner; however he did show communicative gestures towards mother in limited quality and quantity when needing help. In place of gestures and verbal speech, he would place the mother's hand on an object or place the object in the mother's hand with communicative intent for her to help.

During this assessment, she observed his eye contact, play-based abilities, and repetitive behavior typically associated with his Autism Spectrum Disorder.

Chapter 2: Raising Jiraiya

Jiraiya has always held great eye contact. That was something that caused confusion about the autism diagnosis for me. I had always believed that kids with autism were unable to maintain good eye contact with others.

> Behaviorally, Jiraiya demonstrated some repetitive play behaviors, including continuous pressing of buttons on the toy and the music box and repeating this over and over until the object was removed. Jiraiya displayed unusual sensory interest during the observation (e.g., feeling objects by rubbing hands slowly over them, examining toys visually, and hand/finger twisting closely in front of eyes, and putting bubbles to mouth when popping them.)

She then explained that Jiraiya was on the Autism spectrum and diagnosed him as having Autism Spectrum Disorder (ASD), Level 3.

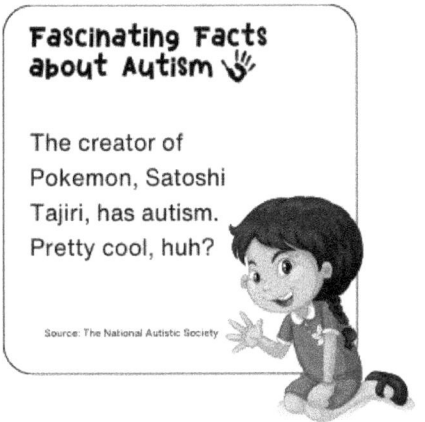

Fascinating Facts about Autism

The creator of Pokemon, Satoshi Tajiri, has autism. Pretty cool, huh?

Source: The National Autistic Society

As a mom, this was all new information for me, so I wanted to take this time to share this with you, as a great resource. Take notice of any familiar behaviors you may have observed with your child. It's not about being in fear, but being aware and taking early intervention action.

According to Autism Speaks, the following table shows the different levels and behavioral traits.

Table 1: Severity Levels for Autism Spectrum Disorder

Severity level	Social communication	Restricted, repetitive behaviors
Level 3 Requiring very substantial support	Severe deficits in verbal and nonverbal social communication skills cause severe impairments in functioning, very limited initiation of social interactions, and minimal response to social overtures from others. For example, a person with few words of intelligible speech who rarely initiates interaction and, when he or she does, makes unusual approaches to meet needs only and responds to only very direct social approaches	Inflexibility of behavior, extreme difficulty coping with change, or other restricted/repetitive behaviors markedly interfere with functioning in all spheres. Great distress/difficulty changing focus or action.

Chapter 2: Raising Jiraiya

Level 2 Requiring substantial support	Marked deficits in verbal and nonverbal social communication skills; social impairments apparent even with supports in place; limited initiation of social interactions; and reduced or abnormal responses to social overtures from others. For example, a person who speaks simple sentences, whose interaction is limited to narrow special interests, and how has markedly odd nonverbal communication.	Inflexibility of behavior, difficulty coping with change, or other restricted/repetitive behaviors appear frequently enough to be obvious to the casual observer and interfere with functioning in a variety of contexts. Distress and/or difficulty changing focus or action.
Level 1 Requiring support	Without supports in place, deficits in social communication cause noticeable impairments. Difficulty initiating social interactions, and clear examples of atypical or unsuccessful response to social overtures of others. May appear to have decreased interest in social interactions. For example, a person who is able to speak in full sentences and engages in communication but whose to- and-fro conversation with others fails, and whose attempts to make friends are odd and typically unsuccessful.	Inflexibility of behavior causes significant interference with functioning in one or more contexts. Difficulty switching between activities. Problems of organization and planning hamper independence.

It was what I expected to hear, and I now had a game plan on what needed to be done. The idea of the "label" is controversial amongst some families and individuals. According to an article on Spark for Autism,

> Around the world, many societies view autism as a source of disappointment, annoyance, or shame. According to some researchers, this social stigma may keep families from seeking a diagnosis and services for their children, participating fully in their communities, and enjoying the same quality of life as their neighbors. Stigma may affect an autistic person's ability to make friends, date, and get or keep a job. Some adults even worry about telling their doctors that they have autism.

I have even heard parents of students I previously taught say they didn't want their child to be labeled because they feared it would create more issues than interventions could remedy. They believed their child would be treated differently and not have fair or equal opportunities.

I wanted the diagnosis for Jiraiya because I felt it opened up more doors to the help we needed than the suspicion ever would. I was able to have him referred to specialists who were able to help him communicate better and learn to cope with self-regulatory behaviors.

He had IEPs and 504s in school that provided accommodations to help him achieve and become his best self. I never cared what the world thought of him; that didn't matter to me. I only cared about being his mom, and I knew that no amount of embarrassment or socially unacceptable behavior would keep me from helping him the way he needed the help.

The diagnosis from the LMFT happened in February 2020, right before COVID-19 hit. He would do a half day (2 hours) at a local early childhood school, where I began teaching that year.

The program is called Early Childhood Special Education (ESCE). This would be good to help him socialize and learn routines. Then, in March 2020, as we all know, the world shut down. I tried to work with Jiraiya on Zoom meetings he would have with his school, but it was tough to get him to focus, so we did what we could during the day.

We waited almost a year to be seen by the Developmental Pediatrician. The referral was placed in June 2019, and his appointment to see Jiraiya's development pediatrician was in June 2020. He was now 3 1 2 years old.

During the time we waited, his sleep was almost non-existent. For years, I had put Jiraiya down for bed at 8 p.m., but despite the consistency in routine, he wouldn't fall asleep. Not only would he not fall asleep at 8 p.m., but he wouldn't stay asleep through the night.

Most of our nights ended at 11 p.m., and the next day usually started around 2 or 3 in the morning! I was exhausted, to say the least. It was like having a newborn for years and years. His Primary Care Physician told me that she could not prescribe anything for sleep until he was seen by his Developmental Pediatrician.

I had already received the autism diagnosis, as I previously wrote about, so I had no doubts that Jiraiya would have the same diagnosis. We went in and met with Jiraiya's development pediatrician.

There wasn't much more to the appointment than discussing what I saw at home. He also observed

Jiraiya and his play and interaction. I shared about his sleep patterns or lack thereof.

I was previously advised to give him melatonin; although I did, it did nothing for him. Jiraiya's development pediatrician prescribed him a medication called Clonidine. We started at the lowest dosage, and that night, when he went to sleep. It was as if my prayers had been answered! He fell asleep. It was such a relief.

A NEW DAWN

Jiraiya's development pediatrician prescribed medication and therapy sessions to help with Jiraiya's developmental delays. I was given a list of local Applied Behavioral Analysis (ABA), and Speech Therapy and Occupational Therapy clinics. I called, and some of the wait lists in the area were over a year long!

But let me digress a minute to explain ABA - these terms can get confusing.

According to an article by Autism Speaks, *ABA is a therapy based on the science of learning and behavior.*

It is typically used to help people with autism and other developmental disorders learn behaviors that help them live safer and more fulfilling lives.

ABA focuses on teaching necessary skills and stopping dangerous behaviors rather than preventing harmless self-stimulatory behavior (stims).

Therapists work with autistic people to improve skills like:

- Communication and language abilities
- Social skills
- Self-care and hygiene routines
- Play and leisure skills
- Motor abilities

The goal is not for someone to appear neurotypical but for their lives to be improved in a way that is meaningful to them.

In the fall of 2020, Jiraiya was enrolled in a local daycare program. Jim and I were currently in the middle of our custody battle. When Jiraiya attended the daycare, it was only for a half day. The first half of the day was spent in an ESCE program at the local early childhood school. They would bus him to the

Chapter 2: Raising Jiraiya

daycare when the day ended, and he would stay there until I picked him up after work.

The woman who would be his caretaker, I'll call her Ms. Janine, seemed very nice. She was very helpful. During the day, I received a phone call asking if there was anything she needed to know about Jiraiya. This was code for, *I've noticed he's autistic but don't know how to ask more directly, so I'll ask in a roundabout way.*

I told her that Jiraiya was diagnosed with autism. However, I was sure I had told them before because he was enrolled in a Special Education Program at my school, and they would drop him off.

She assured me that Jiraiya was in good hands because she was a mother of a child with autism. Any worry that I had immediately disappeared. You can have a heart for children with special needs, but I believe it becomes more instinctual when you have your own child with special needs.

For example, I see my son in all children with special needs. I think about how I would want someone to treat my son. I absolutely adore him, and it hurts me sometimes when people stare at him when he's trying to regulate his body in ways that are not socially acceptable. Still, he's not harming anyone; if it brings him comfort, that should be the most important thing.

Unfortunately, others do not share the same sentiment. For example, one day we were inside a store, and there were a lot of people. He must have been overwhelmed and had difficulty regulating his emotions, so when I asked him to "come here," he shrieked at the highest pitched ever, "Commmmeee heeeeeere." A little girl, about 10 years old, covered her ears and said, "Gosh," while glaring at Jiraiya.

I apologized and told her he didn't mean to hurt her ears. If you ever want to be a supportive person to a special needs parent, don't stare at the child. Take the time to explain to your own child about children with special needs or say some children need extra help.

Either way, back to the daycare worker. I started getting more notifications when I picked Jiraiya up that he had started acting out. He was hitting, kicking, and running around the classroom. I believed that he was running around the classroom thing... I was more hesitant to believe that he was being aggressive.

He was with an excellent stay-at-home sitter for the first 3 years of his life, and I had never heard any complaints about him. Of course, she said the usual... that he was very active, but if you know Jiraiya, that sums up who he is in a nutshell. He has more energy than anyone I have ever known. He has more energy than anyone I will ever know.

Something wasn't making sense. I thought about what could be causing the increase in aggression. I hadn't changed anything in my house. I wasn't harsh with Jiraiya. I don't raise my voice, and I don't spank him. I don't believe using these forms of discipline would be helpful for him because of his level of cognition.

He might understand how I was feeling or how it made him feel because of his ability to understand energies. He wouldn't understand why I was being mean to him. I was his safe person and wanted to always be that for him.

However, his dad was a government contractor and had just returned from another overseas assignment. He hadn't been around Jiraiya in a few months, who had just turned 4.

His dad firmly believes in the "spare the rod, spoil the child" philosophy. I didn't see it until it was too late, and when I decided to have a child with him, I thought I could always protect my child from the tantrums that his father would take out on his children.

Never did I think I would be unable to protect him. I heard later that Jiraiya started receiving corporal punishment and verbal rages beginning at the age of 2 years.

Could you imagine? An autistic 2-year-old in fight or flight because his dad was unable to control his impulses and wanted so badly to control a child, who at this time was unable to control his own body.

I remember a phone call I received on May 5, 2021. It was from Jiraiya's dad's ex-wife. She called me, and I immediately sensed the desperation in her voice. She asked me where Jiraiya was as if to try to make sense of something and establish his safety. I told her he was with his dad, and she immediately told me how worried she was. She had just gotten off the phone with her son, Jiraiya's brother, who was tricked into living with his dad while his mom moved to a different state by some strange case of deceit.

She told me that she heard Jim yelling very aggressively and a child in the background incoherently crying and repeating everything said as if to appease the person yelling at him. I knew immediately that this was Jiraiya. He was 4 then and still had minimal communication, including echolalia or parroting what he heard.

Chapter 2: Raising Jiraiya

I asked, "What can I do?" The woman who called me said she didn't want communication to be cut off from her son. She said that if Jiraiya's dad found out, she told me she wouldn't be able to speak to her son. I didn't want that to happen and didn't know what to do, so I did nothing. I will never make that mistake again.

Thinking back to what I could have done differently, I should have called the cops. I should have emailed his dad. I should have tried to help my baby, who was so confused and helpless about why he was treated this way. I felt absolutely trapped in that decision, and I regret that tremendously.

However, his school started noticing the difference in aggressive behavior. At first, it would be a small topic of conversation when I picked him up from the daycare. They would mention something that he had done, and hours had passed by the time I picked him up. I would apologize, but at that time, Jiraiya had no concept of time and didn't remember what he had done.

He couldn't explain why he felt compelled to act the way he had. I didn't harp on it because if Jiraiya was not corrected at that moment, then it wouldn't really do anything for him if I talked about it four hours later.

At this time, Jiraiya did not have the cognition or self-awareness to reflect on his behaviors. They were impulses that were acted upon to get what he wanted. We were working on his ability to answer yes/no questions, so asking him to respond to an earlier incident had no effect because he was unable to self-reflect.

Then, the complaints became daily, almost as if they were fed up with dealing with him. I felt so bad I would go during my conference and try to help out in any way I could. I would notice that when I would enter his classroom, he was usually kept to himself. While the other kids played at stations, he usually sat at a table, and there was no one to sit and interact with. I tried to get him to interact with the others to help him feel more comfortable. I would introduce him to the other kids and show interest in their toys.

It seems as if the daycare workers didn't want to do anything that would actually help Jiraiya. They just wanted him to sit at a table and do nothing more to help. On one occasion, when all the other kids were going to the potty, they didn't ask Jiraiya if he needed to go. At this time, he was still not potty trained and

Chapter 2: Raising Jiraiya

was 4 ½. They said they did not ask him because it would embarrass him.

If you know anything about children with autism, they are not easily embarrassed. Their diagnosis is a blessing and a curse in this way. That is why they feel no shame stimming in public or asking questions that might seem embarrassing to some. Their social cues do not behave the way that ours does. Part of the DSM-V criteria for autism is social impairments that could affect his ability to interact with others.

I wanted to discuss the severity of what was happening with Jiraiya at the daycare center. The way he was handling corrections and the way he was interacting with other kids. I tried to help them understand his triggers or words/reactions that would send him into chaos.

One of the words was "no". He wanted to be able to do what he wanted, so when he heard "no," he would usually respond by hitting, biting, or screaming at whoever was around. I suggested they not say "no" but use redirection to get him to do what was wanted, but not in a way that would create more turmoil for him and those around him.

I also told them that it was best to start Jiraiya there earlier in the day so that he would only be there in the morning before the bus would take him to Belton Early Childhood School (BECS).

The daycare providers also felt this was best since the childcare provider was consistently there in the morning instead of the afternoon, when sometimes subs were called in while she picked up her child.

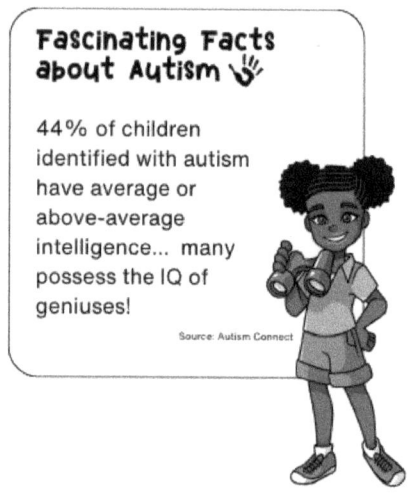

A few weeks later, I received a subpoena that the director and the daycare provider at this local daycare would be testifying on behalf of the father.

Chapter 2: Raising Jiraiya

They would attest that Jiraiya was better behaved when Jim was around and that he was the one who taught them how to speak to him sternly. They said that it seemed to turn everything around for them whenever Jim made these suggestions. They also claimed that I had told the caregivers that Jiraiya was not to be spoken the word "no" and that he was allowed to do whatever he wanted.

I was in disbelief. These people who had promised me they would do everything for my child would now testify against me. The people I conferenced with and sat with daily during my conference time to create a team to help my child had turned their back on me and agreed that Jiraiya was "better behaved" when he was in the presence of his dad. They didn't recognize his behavior for what it was: fear. Jiraiya was terrified of his father.

Following this awareness, I received a phone call that Jiraiya had broken Mrs. Janine's glasses from hitting her. His dad was called but didn't want to take off work to investigate the problem, so I went there immediately.

Upon walking in, I was directed over to the church's sanctuary. What I saw immediately enraged me. The class was on the stage, practicing for an upcoming spring recital. I looked over, and Jiraiya was off stage by himself. He made a noise and was yanked over to Ms. Janine, who clearly had lost her patience. Jiraiya immediately began yelling and I started to walk over there because who in their right mind yanks a child with special needs?!

I was distraught, and I was having a hard time remaining calm after what I saw. I started talking to the director and the daycare worker. I was then told how they were unequipped to handle Jiraiya. They didn't have the equipment they needed, nor did they have the training.

This is an issue that I believe we, as autistic families must face, it is challenging to find understanding and compassionate caregivers who are willing to work with our children.

A couple hours later, I received a phone call stating that Jiraiya would be placed on "administrative leave" since they could no longer "handle" him. Fortunately, I had a family friend willing to care for Jiraiya for about 3 hours in the morning before the school bus picked him up at 10:30 to take him to school.

During that time, I would get daily notifications or photos about how Jiraiya's day was going. I would hear about the things he would do and the foods he

Chapter 2: Raising Jiraiya

ate, but most importantly, Jiraiya was working on potty training. He went to the potty every 10 minutes. The friend who was watching Jiraiya explained to Jiraiya what was happening and would make it a ritual to flush the toilet and wash his hands after going to the bathroom. After two weeks, Jiraiya was fully potty trained and did not need to wear pull-ups anymore.

Jiraiya's ad litem knew of an ABA place because her neighbor's son had attended. We contacted the facility director at the local ABA clinic,, and she scheduled an appointment for observation to see if this would benefit Jiraiya. The meeting lasted about an hour, and she asked my concerns and what was happening in his life. She asked us to leave so that she could do a complete evaluation of Jiraiya so he was not in the presence of a parent.

I came back an hour later, and the facility director had noticed the attention-seeking behaviors that he was exhibiting. She said he attempted to bite her, not out of frustration but more because he wanted a reaction. I thought back to the daycare, and every time I would visit him, he was sitting at a table all by himself. There was a constant complaint from the daycare providers that he would bite, but it seemed he was really seeking attention; he didn't have the language to say this.

She recommended that Jiraiya begin ABA therapy. Of course, due to insurance, we had to wait about a week before he could start. The ABA therapy would replace the daycare, and he would stay there during the day while I was at work.

ABA THERAPY BEGINS

I dropped Jiraiya off on a Monday, a little fearful and nervous. I was so used to how things had been at the daycare that I immediately started going down the list of looks for triggers, how quickly I could be there, etc.

The facility director looked at me and said, "Mom, we got this. That's why you're bringing him to us." Immediately, I exhaled the breath I had been holding, smiled, and said, "Ok, I will see y'all at 4 o'clock." It was a relief to have someone willing to work with Jiraiya and someone I could trust.

ABA has been such a relief to my family. Jiraiya's inconsistent care at a daycare setting was horrendous and not helpful for him or his diagnosis. He would become easily upset, and it was apparent that the people caring for him were not interested in giving him the quality of care required for a young child with his diagnosis.

Currently, Jiraiya attends daily Monday-Friday from 8 a.m.-4 p.m. They continue to work on his communication skills, among other things, as noted earlier. We continue to take him to Speech Therapy and Occupation Therapy twice weekly in addition to the ABA therapy that he receives 5 days a week.

He is currently kindergarten-aged, but I am looking to begin the evaluation process because he will enter 1st grade next year, which will look different because he is required to attend school at this age.

Me and his father went to court in November of 2021, a month before Jiraiya turned 5. In this meeting, we had agreed to a settlement. Although I didn't feel it was in Jiraiya's best interest to have a 50/50 custody split, I thought I was the only person looking out for Jiraiya's need for consistency.

His father and ad-litem said that he should be able to go back and forth between households, week-on-week off, but we would switch between homes on Wednesday nights.

The behavior that followed this agreement was one that I had anticipated. Jiraiya showed more aggression and more self-stimulating behaviors, such as arm flapping, finger twirling, and vocal stims. When his ABA therapist suggested that we not do the Wednesday overnights at the other parent's house and stay at one parent's house for a week, we saw a decrease in aggression.

I have unfortunately been undermined in several decisions regarding Jiraiya since the agreement. His father doesn't see consistency as important as I do. Jiraiya's schedule while with his dad is very sporadic, and some days/weeks, he doesn't attend at all. Sometimes, Jim will ask for medication for Jiraiya without consulting me. Then, Jiraiya's medication adversely affects his behavior.

I cannot stress this enough: if you are co-parenting with another adult to care for your autistic child, you both need to be on the same page and follow the advice of developmental pediatricians, behavioral therapists, speech therapists, and occupational therapists. Do not act out of spite towards the other parent; do what is best for your child, who is already fighting a battle we know little about.

YOU ARE NOT ALONE

I have learned so much from being an autism mom. I have learned patience and how to be my child's advocate because, at this point in time, I am his voice.

My job is to ensure he is successful, confident, and, most importantly, loved. I believe my life's mission is to help him be the most successful version of himself. I will not rest until I know that he is either able to care for himself or that he can advocate to get the help that he needs.

It is also my life's mission to bring public awareness and let others know that you are not in this alone. Autism Awareness is essential, but more than that, what do we do with that awareness? How do we include those who carry that diagnosis? How do we support the families of children with this life-long disability? It's not an easy road, and I know it firsthand.

There are many resources available for children with autism. Some are entirely free and can create lifelong advantages for your child. If you suspect your child might have the diagnosis, please take the first step.

Take your child to their pediatrician and discuss your concerns. There are steps your child's pediatrician will take if they suspect there is a developmental delay. Ask your pediatrician to refer your child for speech therapy, occupational therapy, and/or ECI, as well as a developmental pediatrician who will be able to make the official autism diagnosis.

You can call ECI independently, without a doctor's referral, as they are a community outreach program. They will provide an evaluation and prescribe further services, most free or low-cost, to the families. Early intervention is essential and makes a world of difference for your child.

Also, look into local foundations that can sponsor children and their families. Many therapies can be costly, requiring crazy out-of-pocket costs and deductibles. I have found a local non-profit organization, Imagine A Way. This non-profit is a central Texas-based charity.

> Imagine A Way stands in the gap for families that have a child on the autism spectrum in need of critical therapeutic services. Therapies in the preschool years make the most significant impact on a child's lifelong success. We help

children with autism get the help they need during the years they need it most.

I would highly recommend looking into their resources if you need help or donating to their wonderful organization if you're able. They have supported my family by offering insurance to Jiraiya to cover his ABA therapy and pay out-of-pocket costs for ABA, Speech therapy, occupational therapy, and developmental pediatrician visits.

Go to www.imagineaway.org to check out resources for your specific needs.

A GLIMMER OF HOPE

Update: As of May 31, 2023, Jiraiya no longer attends ABA because he has regressed and was unable to make progress. He also no longer attends speech or OT.

However, I am trying to get him back in because the other household, where he stayed 50% of the time, did not take him to the appointments when he was staying at their house. I have also received my real estate license so that I can have a more flexible schedule for him and help other parents with special needs.

I am also continuing to teach. Jiraiya will attend school in an autism program called Elements, which is very similar to an ABA setting.

So how do I know I'm on the right path? I will quote Ralph Waldo Emerson on his poem titled "What is Success":

> "To appreciate beauty;
> To find the best in others;
> To give of one's self;
> To leave the world a bit better, whether by a healthy child, a garden patch, or a redeemed social condition."

I will continue to try to make the world a little bit better by the children that I raise. I hope that by hearing my story, it brought comfort and hope. I hope that this inspires you to be the voice for your child. I hope you are able to look at my experience and see what steps you can take to help your child, wherever they're at, and that you are not alone.

Chapter 2: Raising Jiraiya

Don't forget about yourself in this process. Take care of yourself. If you would like to reach out with questions, concerns, or would like someone to listen to your story, feel free to contact me via email:

melesiahudson0811@gmail.com.

Now get ready for a lot of dose of cuteness! My heart revealed on the next page ♡♡♡ >>>>>>>>>>>>

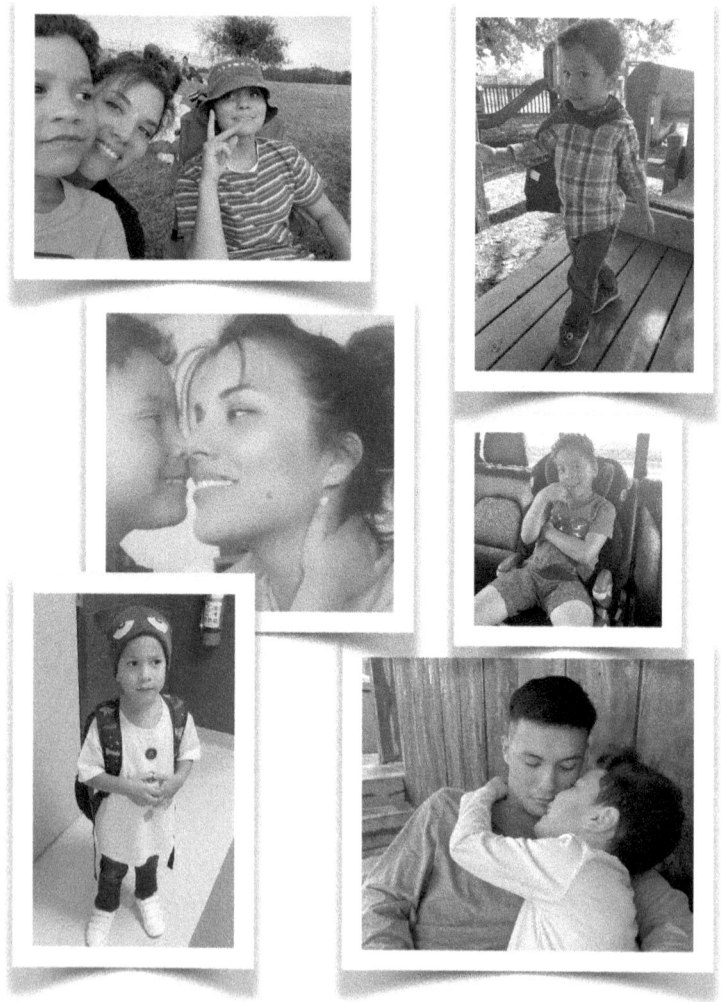

Chapter 2: Raising Jiraiya

LETTERS TO MY BROTHER

To my brother Jiraiya, to whom I love so much. This note is to let you know that if you were to read this in the future, how much you mean to me and what you have taught me through these past 6 years. I am writing this from my heart and to share this with the world.

Patience-You my little brother, have taught me to be patient with you but with other's. You have shown me that not everyone is out to get me. Before, I didn't know how to express myself at time and I now understand I needed to be more patient and understanding. I also feel like this helps with how I interact with others.

Anger-You helped me at a time when I didn't know how to express myself. You have been there when I needed you. I remember a time when I was sad. I was crying and you ran up to me and gave me a hug like you understood. It changed my outlook on life that day.

Future-I think about your future and the future I want for all of us. I want for you to be accepted and not for people to stay away because they think you are weird. I want a future where your condition is not used to describe someone or their limitations.

Instead, it should be seen as the ultimate clean slate and whatever you choose to go after, will be accomplished. I value you and have high hopes for your future.

Love, Mavric

-♡ ♡ ♡-

Jiraiya,

I honestly never thought I would have guess I would get to have a brother with autism. Before I used to think those kids who would scream loudly, randomly were weird and I'd try not to stare at them like everyone else, but after you I realize just how much everyone goes through raising an autistic child, and also how human you are, just like the rest of us.

If there's anything I learned from you, it's that if I have time to judge, I'd rather spend

Chapter 2: Raising Jiraiya

that time learning about the things I don't understand. You do a lot of weird things, like burying yourself in the couch or getting excited over something colorful.

You are also fun to be around, like how you get me excited to go trick-or-treating on Halloween just by flapping your hands and jumping, or how I can talk to you about anything and not feel judged because I know you can hear us, you only choose not to respond.

I like how you get obsessions with the randomest things, like the Five Little Pumpkins or Baby Shark. Or how there are certain foods you love eating and others you refuse to eat. Like who doesn't like jelly on their PBNJ??!

Anyways, I know how people are. There will always be someone who dislikes you. It'll be especially hard because you have autism. People are just going to say mean things and not try to understand what you or everybody around you goes through.

At some point in your life, you may feel loneliness. People may disregard you as autistic and disabled rather than another human being with feelings and things you like and dislike, things you enjoy and people you like being around. I'm sure you feel lonely sometimes.

  That's why I like sitting with you sometimes. I know I would want someone to do the same for me. To make sure I'm feeling ok and seen. If you ever need someone to sit at the table with you, come to me. I'll listen to you how I remember you would listen to me.

—Your only sister, Mikaila

P.S. Jelly is really good, give it a try. :)

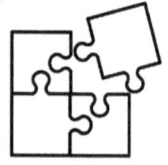

REFERENCES

Center for Disease Control and Prevention article titled-Important Milestones: Your Baby by 15 months, reviewed on December 12, 2022
15 Month Visit -. https://www.laurelwoodpediatrics.com/15-month-visit/

Early Childhood Intervention Services (ECI) | Texas Health and Human Services. https://www.hhs.texas.gov/services/disability/early-childhood-intervention-services?msclkid=58d43efdd07611ec9786ac94aef505e7

Center for Life Resources - ECI - Early Childhood Intervention. https://www.kendallcountygivingconnections.com/organizations/center-for-life-resources---eci---early-childhood-intervention

What is Community-Based Early Intervention?. https://www.appliedbehavioranalysisprograms.com/faq/community-based-early-intervention/?amp=1

SPARK for Autism | The Stigma of Autism: When Everyone is Staring at You. https://wp-demo.sparkforautism.org/stigma-autism/

Questions and Answers About ABA | Autism Speaks. https://www.autismspeaks.org/blog/questions-and-answers-about-aba

Imagine A Way presents 8th Annual Gala - CultureMap Austin. https://austin.culturemap.com/eventdetail/imagine-way-8th-annual-gala

ABOUT THE AUTHOR

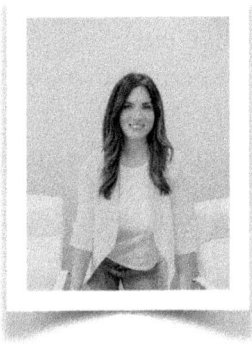

Meet Melesia Hudson, a compassionate 38-year-old teacher and dedicated real estate agent, whose life is a harmonious blend of nurturing three incredible children—Mavric, Mikaila, and Jiraiya.

Graduating from the University of Mary Hardin-Baylor in 2011, Melesia embarked on a journey that seamlessly integrates her roles as an educator, real estate professional, and now, an inspiring author.

In her debut book, Melesia brings her unique perspective and heartfelt dedication to light. With a profound understanding of the challenges faced by families affected by autism, her goal is clear: to extend a helping hand to those navigating the intricate journey of raising a child with autism.

Melesia's narrative transcends the realms of real estate, reaching into the hearts of families, single parents, and siblings, offering a beacon of hope and creating awareness about the nuances of life influenced by autism.

With a fervent passion for connecting families with homes that provide not just shelter but a haven of stability and safety for their loved ones with autism, Melesia's mission is to foster a sense of belonging and support. Her book is a testament to her commitment to creating more opportunities, understanding, and empathy for families traversing the unique landscape of autism.

Through her writing, Melesia aspires to be a catalyst for positive change, shedding light on the challenges, triumphs, and untold stories within the realm of autism. Join her on this journey of compassion, awareness, and advocacy, as she strives to make a lasting impact in the lives of those touched by autism.

Chapter 2: Raising Jiraiya

"

We were never meant to heal alone!
– msMISSYms

Chapter 3

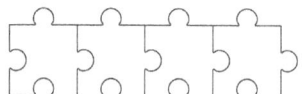

The Neurodi-Way by msMISSYms

Counseling is fun, especially when many of the *"I don't want to talk about these emotions"* topic(s) can be treated or regulated by oneself with an easy-to-learn and apply *brain hack*.

Counselors are professionally trained language artisans who facilitate counseling skills while engaging with their client in the art and science called Mental Health Therapy, which, like engineering, is an applied science.

A counselor, like most artists, may or may not choose to blend psychology theories, culture, spirituality, neuroscience, research, and their client's lived experiences into their therapeutic process -- almost similar to a painter's instinctive choice in their selection of a tool, theory, inspiration, etc. to not take their purpose to act or to not act while they paint.

The success and joy I witness in my clients have inspired me to reexamine trauma treatment approaches. I am proud to report I, too, changed during the COVID-19 pandemic in 2021, and so has the manner in which I define myself.

I am more than a chronic pain patient; I am a mother, a friend, a wife, a world citizen, and professionally I am a mind-body psychotherapist. My life's purpose today is to pay the kindness bestowed upon me during more than a decade of personal study to heal myself forward to the community of my youth as an advocate for any initiative that promotes a personal responsibility message for each member of society to learn/practice/brain hack ANS (autonomic nervous system) techniques.

Don't worry, I'll explain :) Let me introduce to you a term I coined myself (and also the title of my chapter): The Neurodi-Way

The Neurodi-Way phrase is a fun, positive, identity-affirming name I made up for the Attention-deficit/hyperactivity disorder (ADHD) and Autism

Neurodivergent client population's brain hacks that I smashed up to facilitate trauma interventions over the internet during the pandemic shutdown.

Quick to learn, engaging, and un-shaming, the Neruodi-Way phrase itself has redefined 'different' as not at all equal to being disabled. If I could, I would and/or should diagnose normalcy as a disabled concept. Normalcy requires "a pride-of-oneself" to want to engage in the internal realms of one's mind and body to learn about oneself so one can be oneself in a world that can be very confusing and shaming to us all.

Had it not been for the courage of my autistic clients, many of whom are young teens, I'd be likely to still believe I must continue to *fix* myself. Therefore, with your permission and because my girlfriend asked me, I am sharing the "brain hack smash-ups" my clients shared as the best "calmers" to come out of the pandemic's unique therapeutic environment pressure that challenged all mental health providers.

With heartfelt humility, I will share an easy-to-facilitate self-practice program because I was asked for my assistance to face a challenging systemic issue of our time: emotional dysregulation.

My goal is to offer my community affordable access to some of the best therapeutic trauma treatment approaches I have personally experienced and may facilitate in my practice. If the concepts of the Neurodi-Way inspired approach are successful, we will all know it because the self-regulation of one's ANS is empowering and will, I hope, lead to each of us living/being oneself from a place of self-peace—which to me is world peace.

BRAIN HACK EXPLAINED

Once I agreed to write this chapter, my common-sense thinking mindset said to self, "I better take a few more classes"... one being Dr. Ganty's certified clinical trauma practitioner.

Dr. Ganty's brain hack, Noodling, is a fabulous technique to start the chapter. Noodling as a brain hack concept exemplifies well the power of our mind-body connection. It gives us a better understanding of how our thoughts about ourselves are shaped by our unconscious survival instincts, and how these two aspects can affect each other.

There are many researchers to thank for their dedication to psychology and their efforts to raise the money required to research the many interventions I love to smash-up.

For example, in Dr. Ganty's innovative approach, there are elements from various techniques like self-directed neuroplasticity, self-hypnosis, mindfulness, brainspotting, somatic experiencing, and somatic psychology theory.

These methods quickly help you focus on becoming aware of tension in your muscles. Dr. Ganty's unique method, using an analogy-style approach, makes it easy for clients to understand and remember. It's a safe and practical way for clients to use on their own when needed.

A brain that fears often likely has a trauma history. I have heard more than once my favorite trauma expert, Dr. Peter Levin, emphasize that if there is trauma, there is amnesia. Therefore, amnesia is one tool the ANS utilizes to protect the mind from the recall of past painful "situations."

To protect us from remembering painful experiences, our brains evolved to separate our current sense of self from past thoughts, symbols, memories, and so on. This self-preservation mechanism is a bit like strict discipline in parenting.

It may seem helpful in the short term for managing immediate situations, but research shows that frequent use can lead to long-term negative consequences that can affect our performance in personal and professional relationships.

These consequential feelings are a self-created sense of fear that is often just a "recalled felt" feeling within the body and can become overwhelming, even more so to a brain with any learning processing delay(s), which adds to the complexity of writing treatment plans to treat the anxiety symptoms of children who identify as Autistic and/or ADHD, Neurodivergent.

Dr. Ganty's trauma therapy brain hack, in my opinion, is a really cool ANS self-mood-regulator, too, as it is helpful for anyone who experiences anxiety due to any perceived or misperceived notion of even just the slightest possibility that it is conceivable to believe any past unsatisfied memory, real or imagined, will repeat itself again.

So, whenever something like a thought, conversation, or even a background song reminds you of past disappointments or a lack of self-confidence, which can trigger old painful memories or physical discomfort like stomachaches, your body's automatic response system will do whatever it takes to prevent those feelings from coming back.

Words you might hear your child speak, if applicable to monitor your child for an anxiety disorder, are statements like "I didn't mean to" or "I don't know" (a great answer, too, by the way).

The fear of repeating mistakes is a major concern for many children who identify as 'different' especially from their neuro-typical peers. It is impossible to talk oneself out of a fear state because the physical and mental state of the body is chemically composed and involuntarily activated to fuel a body's state of anxiety/panic to address any perceived threat stressor.

Hence, prevention is a skill-enrichment resource, an essential trauma-informed measure for all counselors to self-practice and advocate.

The anxiety we feel is often caused by our own tensing, quick movements, or self-imposed stress, as our body tries to either escape or face a challenge. These anxious feelings are linked to both our mental and physical state.

When our body senses that a situation has crossed a personal or societal boundary we've set, it can go to extreme lengths to protect us, even if it means cutting off blood supply to our thinking brain. This tricks us into thinking that disconnecting from the pain response is the safest option, even when healthier connections with ourselves and others are available.

It is important to note that the body holds *stress chemicals* within the cells from past traumatic experiences that lend to the body's ability to develop muscle memory reflexes to implicit memories--the longest held-on-to memories stored in the mind-body.

Think of riding a bike. You do not have to relearn nor think about how to balance yourself every time you ride a bike, regardless of how much time has passed once you master the skill.

It is, for this reason, the many intrusive or unwanted behaviors that challenge people during their lifetime are often old implicit (muscle) memories developed by our nervous systems as a solution for any misunderstood or difficult challenge(s) experienced by each of us within our non-verbal years, otherwise known as, the child's neurodevelopmental years of brain development.

For this reason, no person's response to a traumatic event can be compared to another's. The environments our brains all developed within are so exponentially different that an individual's trauma history, even amongst twins, is as unique as a fingerprint.

The importance of tracking one's own body tension is then a necessary mind-body preventative measure to prevent oneself from being triggered to, for example, maybe hit or verbally abuse another or oneself.

Noodling's brain hack entails an internal focus of the mind's eye on one's tense muscles. Once the mind identifies the felt sense of tension, the client imagines wiggling noodles in their muscle(s) until the tension is released.

A Neurodi smash-up to add-on to this hack is to color in the noodles with any color one's imagination chooses to represent their act of kindness towards oneself, which provides the mind the opportunity to comfort the body with self-empathy for the much effort required by oneself to manage the stress most often caused by what happened to the self in its past and is not necessarily the fault of oneself.

Therefore, noodle your tense muscles when you or your child is fidgety. It is an act of self-compassion and care that requires maintenance, like brushing your teeth. Wiggle wiggle wiggle then throughout your day, every day, to track how much tension you hold in your body daily and discover how it influences your reactions to stressors.

A core therapeutic construct of each of my smash-ups derives from an Acceptance and Compassion Therapy (ACT) approach. Children can focus only on one emotion's existence within their mind's awareness of their present known sense of oneself.

If your child has a negative mindset, then it is likely your child will not believe a compliment, even if it was observed by the caregiver as appreciated by their child.

I have noticed with my clients that pulling apart the 'black/white thinking' into 'shades of grey thinking' can be distressing for them--as it is difficult for a Neurodivergent—since the many grey "situations" can start to feel overwhelming.

Therefore, I instruct my clients to be fair to themselves like the client would want to be represented in a court of law. If the child is only stating their negative side of the story to themselves but would criticize a lawyer if their positive side was not represented, I ask my clients if it is fair to do it to themselves? Otherwise, the sense of self's protector of fairness, anger, will be angry at one's self.

The Neurodi-Way is a kind approach that offers verbal and nonverbal Neurodi, an alternative to talk therapy. Achieving peace of mind through brain hacking is a self-directed response. To do so, one must first overcome the internal barriers that prevent trusting the brain's purpose. This process involves calculating the risks associated with a neuro-diverse mind filled with many unknowns.

The hack then is a contracted trust between the brain and the mind to source work out to the brain to do the calculations of the many grey-area thinking for the "it depends on the situation" memories cause, hey, the brain can calculate the variables of each memory much more quickly.

So, trust your brain, trust the process, and you never know until you try; you might trust yourself as there is no right or wrong way, so have fun and make it your own.

Now, the Neurodi community has a straightforward technique to boost confidence in their ability to make decisions while remaining calm. This approach helps them when a situation arises, and they need to choose whether to react or not.

It's a much-needed alternative to the endless pondering and overthinking that many Neurodi individuals experience daily, as they often obsess over the potential risks and what-ifs.

The share I kindly offer now back to the Neurodi community also documents my clients' shared success—I name it "the Neurodi-Way."

Plus, thank you to my town's code officer; I have chosen to serve these loopholes daily as my storefront's product to serve my customers and community in every cup of curiosity six days a week.

Thank you to outside-the-box thinking, as brain hacks are now metaphorically brewed daily in every smashed-up brain hack cup of loopholes for the Neurodi and the neurotypical populations at my new storefront's, trauma prevention and generalized ANS treatment approach facility I call my "Mental Health Loopholes Café: the House of Neurodi and Home to ALL Deer-Me Believers."

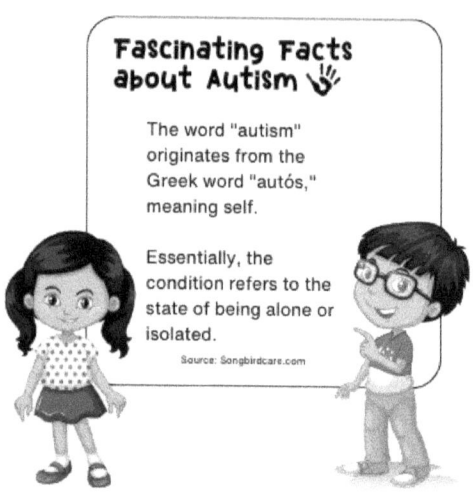

SMASH-UPS & DEER ME EXPLAINED

I first wrote Deer-Me for myself and a friend to share the message I was taught by nature while I observed a trapped, injured deer in my backyard, which I later named Houdini.

Without my knowledge at the time, the same brain hacks I learned as I trained to become a trauma therapist, I found to be notably like the steps I wrote as I chronologized the miracle I witnessed and wrote about many years prior.

Chapter 3: The Neurodi-Way

> To read the Deer Me allegory, please visit my website at www.emotionallyrewired.com—it is presented in its original first draft format, without copywriting or trademarks, because it was, I believe, always intended to be shared.

During the pandemic, the allegory known as 'Deer-Me' transformed into a tale of hope. As a fellow Neurodivergent, I often shared this story with my community. It felt only natural to incorporate the 'Deer Me' story into my counseling approach, using it as a way to connect with others from different backgrounds.

This decision led me to experiment with indirect-brainspotting interventions, ultimately reshaping my therapeutic focus toward promoting, creating, and facilitating trauma prevention and self-regulation skills.

With great pride, I accept this honor to write about the smash-ups that I and my Neurodi clients created together that, in some reversed direction of fate, also ended my own struggle of eighteen years living in chronic pain.

The smash-up consists of Brainspotting (BSP), hypnotherapy, mindfulness heart-connection to self, the counseling skill of confrontation, and msMISSYms special sauce, Deer Me's reverse direction.

The child places one hand out to their side for the negative belief, saying 'bad,' and then takes their other hand out to the other side of the body to represent the opposing belief, saying 'good.'

The purpose is for the eye to follow the peripheral field of vision to scoop up the seen and unseen brainspots (in the subcortical brain) to include all the child's known sense of being bad and felt sense of being good memories, which is fair to the child's brain and not directed by the therapist's concept of fair.

The child then moves their hands at whatever speed the child prefers until they clap them together in front of their face to represent honor to themselves, as a whole person made up of many parts of self, as a now smashed-up belief.

Thus, the creation of meaning means that the two parts of self, good/bad, belong within the child's mindset. The child then moves their now observed prayer hands (archetype cultural integration) toward their heart space, the truth of one's intention (NeuroAffective Relational Model: NARM).

A *kindness-pause* may be added at this time if one thinks it is useful before speaking to oneself about their intention, direct suggestion: "the truth is somewhere in-between" or "the decision will be made known in the present time."

The *kindness-pause* is a self-care tip I learned from my cohort colleague, mediation instructor Simer, during the NARM 1 training I recently completed. Even though the kindness-pause is not a smash-up, it demonstrates the importance of listening to and then adopting shares from others into meaning-making development.

The purpose of the share was to inform the cohort's leader to pause between teaching modules so each cohort member could take a moment to collect their thoughts and transition their mind and body to the new environment.

I was so touched by the 'kindness-to-self' the transition pause created within me that I decided to name it a *kindness-pause,* and then shared it with my Neurodi population.

I sometimes see my youngest Neurodi wiggle their bodies as they do this smash-up.

❦

The purpose of testing out or practicing the brain hack is for your brain to hack it, making it your own. The special sauce in the above hack is known in therapy as *self-disclosure*.

I chose to become a therapist after creating an allegorical story before starting my graduate studies. My approach blends a quicker assessment of risks with building self-trust, and I strive to guide clients in transitioning to a state of physical safety.

❦

The intuition and guts of the counselors' work on display are at the core of each brain hack shared. Each brain hack's building materials maintain its structural integrity with evidence-based theories and the American Counseling Association's professional code of ethics that most definitely impacted the design of each hack.

These aspects were engineered like a building is constructed to ensure it is safe, culturally appropriate, and representative of its population and to ensure it was tested to be sturdy enough to withstand the known and unknown tests of time.

Such hope fuels my efforts to try. How many tries are you willing to give yourself as I welcome you now to explore the power of your brain with your mind's curiosity as you edu-guess play around with the smash-ups shared in this chapter?

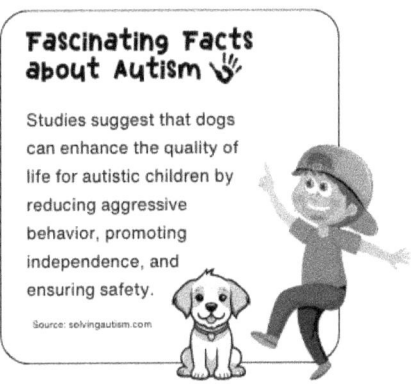

TESTED, TRIED & TRUE - LET'S SMASH-UP!

I encourage you to explore the brain hacks I've created during the pandemic. They're designed to help you uncover and embrace your true self, allowing you to be the best version of yourself while enjoying the process of trying out the following interactive exercises, affectionately known as "smash-ups".

> **Though I am sharing only three in this chapter, visit my website for more Smash-Ups!**

THE PLAYDOUGH SMASH-UP

This brain hack was inspired by brainspotting, holographic color memory, and play therapy:

- Choose a black/white topic that feels comfortable or right. For teaching purposes, the good/bad example used previously will be used throughout the chapter.

Chapter 3: The Neurodi-Way

- Pick the color playdough that represents good for you and place it on a table surface that is OK to play with your playdough.

- Pick the color playdough that represents bad for you and place it on the table.

- The playdough is now in the two appropriate brainspot positions, so begin to look at the two blobs of playdough you placed on the table and notice how you feel.

- As you settle your eye on one color, notice where it is in your body that you feel the sense of it, then slowly move your eye to the next blob of playdough.

- Sit with curiosity about the experience.

- Notice if you are moving your eyes between the two very quickly or slowly

- I welcome you to play with doing the opposite, so if you notice your eyes moving quickly between the two brainspots, then with intention, move your eyes very slowly instead with an open, curious mind; what is it like… difficult> easy> neither?

- At this point, the purpose is for you to keep looking at each spot until they both feel the same. The nervous system is always seeking safety and thus will choose the perceived positive felt sense to regulate itself towards. Oh, did I inform you that this is completely natural for the brain to do...enjoy the process as you observe your inner self's workings like a scientist as you continue to witness with curiosity how your body-mind connection is one.

- Allow for a kind pause for yourself if your child is taking a long time because many Neurodi process deeply, and therefore, they often require longer processing times before they are ready to move on to the next step.

- Once awareness (not perfection) of the felt sense is alike, when you look at each brainspot (playdough), take a piece of the playdough from each and then smash them up together.

- I welcome you to play with noodling here or change lenses.

- Place your awareness on the body's sense of resistance and/or insistence tension.

- Any tension can be pulled by your imagination and your hands as you take pieces from each color and smash them into a new color together.

- A Neurodi smash-up would be to add self-directed hypnosis as one smashes the color of good into the smashed-up color spot: say it is OK to be good and

Chapter 3: The Neurodi-Way

put good into the bad as the bad and good mix the good and bad then gets smashed into the bad. The good goes into the bad, with good mixed up now with the bad to go back into the good, so move the good into the bad.

> The bad with the good now moves to bad, then back into the good as it goes into the bad, and the bad goes into the good. Hence, the good is in the bad, and the bad with good now goes into the good again, but with the good into the bad, and so the bad with good goes back into the good, so the bad is good, and the good is bad, and the bad is good….

- Take the play dough with the new color and make it into any shape you choose, then place the smashed-up color that now represents you as both good and bad with "the truth now is somewhere in-between."

- You can now dry out the playdough shape and place it in your bedroom as your reminder. Make sure to choose a place that feels right; if you cannot find a felt-right place, then ask for a new lens until a felt-sense-of-right is discovered; you must use your internal detective's curiosity eye to find it.

NEW LENSES SMASH-UP

Inspired by Brainspotting, self-hypnosis, direct suggestion, and a Seigel shout-out:

- Sit facing forward, look straight ahead, and think about how good you are.

- Shift your focus from the thoughts of how good you are to your felt-sense in your body of how good you are.

- Does it feel right or off?

- Any part of self that feels off asks with your mind's inner voice the part in the body that is of "new lenses."

- Sit with curiosity as you only observe what is taking place in your body as you say new lenses while still holding the eye position in the forward position.

    This can be tricky, easy, silly, or something you may want to choose to analyze the experience. If you do, are you willing to reverse the direction to decide not to study it?

- If it will be helpful, move your eyes to the right and repeat there and then again on the left.

Chapter 3: The Neurodi-Way

- Remember, not perfection, only introspection (internal awareness with curiosity).

You'd have to be ms MISSY's level of crazy-good curious to try this while looking in the mirror......my husband has his Ph.D. in Organic Chem with research on the mirror image of the carbon atom, which he claims is where drug side effects exist so I thought why not try brainspotting myself in the mirror, it was really cool, that's my share, not clinical advice.

New lenses can be practiced or used whenever something feels "off" in the body while your child is in a new room or just fidgety. A seventeen-year-old female client informed me that her brain hacked this into her own by sharing that she finds herself using it often, self-reported as her fave, whenever she is around people confusing her. It is her kindness-pause to ask herself for a new lens perspective as opposed to just reacting to confusing statements.

According to her, when given direct suggestions for new lenses, she feels calm enough to "reset" herself and ensure that she understands what was said. This enables her to react appropriately within her conception and worldview perspective of an awkward social situation.

A "TIME-IN" LOVE-HUG

A brilliant ACT brain-hack....that's soooo smashable too! This hack comes with a crucial first step...never punish a child for suffering.

- Find a safe space with your child that is not their bed to designate as their time in love hug, just for them only space.

- Stand in the entranceway and have your child look around the room until a space feels right. It may or may not change often, which is fine and is OK to be set up for the child's personal space.

- Put a special blanket, flashlight, and a stuffed animal for the child to hug in the space.

- The stuffed animal is a buddy that requires hugs whenever your child might be feeling like a person you want to punish, so you send them a time-in-love hug instead.

- The child chooses how long the child will need to transfer love and kindness to the stuffed animal until the baby is feeling better.

- When the child is satisfied, the child is to come back and report the good news, which you always celebrate, precisely how you did each time your child stood up when learning to walk.

This brain-hack share is the non-invasive application approach I utilize first to stop children [and an intellectually disabled Autistic non-therapy compliant adult] from biting their caregivers and or harming themselves and or others.

The object offers the child something else to look at in the room to project their shame or blame towards whatever is upsetting the child and it opens naturally a brain-spot for the child to self-process it.

So, if the child's brain chooses to self-brain-spot, you will notice your child sporadically to pause to look at the object curiously whenever it is available to them to view. The purpose of your child self-spotting indirectly is to provide a safe place for your child to shift the discomfort felt in their body more quickly to feel calmer than if the child was instructed only to sit in their room, feeling emotionally pained on their own disconnected from the others.

My journey and professional experiences have led me to a message of empowerment, resilience, and self-discovery. As a Licensed Professional Counselor and

Mind-Body Psychotherapist with specialized certifications in trauma-related therapies, I believe in the power of individuals to take control of their lives, even in the face of adversity.

My commitment to innovative therapeutic solutions, such as founding the Brain-Hack Cafe and working with diverse populations, reflects my dedication to holistic well-being.

I want to emphasize that people have the ability to tap into their inner strengths and make informed choices, embarking on a path of self-discovery, healing, and personal growth.

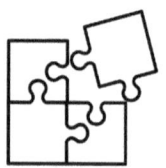

REFERENCES

The Greater Good Magazine, Science-Based Insights for a Meaningful Life
https://greatergood.berkeley.edu

Link to Brainspotting Research and Case Studies
https://brainspotting.com/about-bsp/research-and-case-studies/

Link to Dr. Dan Siegel's Resources Page
https://drdansiegel.com/resources/

msMISSYms website
my website at www.emotionallyrewired.com

ABOUT THE AUTHOR

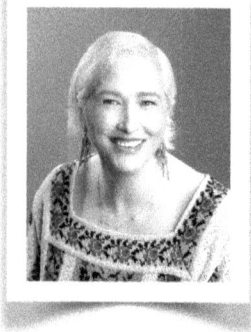

Meet Melissa A. Tatar-Pickersgill, also known as msMISSYms. She identifies as she/her/hers and is a Licensed Professional Counselor and Mind-Body Psychotherapist.

Melissa holds a Master of Science degree in Clinical Mental Health Counseling and is Board Certified as a National Certified Counselor.

She's well-versed in NARM (NeuroAffective Relational Model) and is a Certified Brainspotting Practitioner, along with being a Certified Clinical Trauma Practitioner. To further enhance her expertise, Melissa completed the Certificate in Trauma Stress Studies program at the Trauma Research Center in Boston, MA.

Beyond her contributions at Emotionally Rewired, LLC, Melissa is the visionary behind the Brain-Hack Cafe, established in the spring of 2023. She also dedicates part of her time to working as a Clinician Outpatient Therapist at a behavioral health agency, where she assists children and adults, both with and without Autism and ADHD, ensuring her clearances and insurance are always up to date.

Melissa's journey with Brainspotting began while she was receiving the treatment herself to address grief. This modality proved to be the swiftest and most effective psychotherapeutic tool in her experience, particularly for managing grief and chronic pain.

Having endured chronic pain for more than a decade, Melissa explored numerous treatments following a near-death incident involving an SSRI and muscle relaxer-induced seizure. At that point, medical professionals suggested opioids, physical therapy, and steroid injections as her only path forward.

During her three-day hospital stay, Melissa had a transformative realization and made a deliberate choice. She decided to reclaim her personal power, rejecting fear's influence on her decisions. It was in that hospital bed that she recognized herself as the CEO of her own life for the very first time.

Fascinating Facts about Autism

Those on the autism spectrum often display a natural inclination and talent towards creative pursuits such as music, theater, art, dance, and singing.

Source: Massachusetts General Hospital for Children

Chapter 4

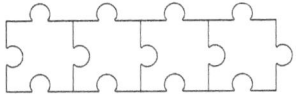

Autism From an Outside Perspective by Evelyn Prewitt

But they that wait upon the Lord shall renew their strength; they shall mount up with wings as eagles; they shall run, and not be weary; and they shall walk, and not faint. -Isaiah 40:31

As I reminisce back to my elementary school days, in the late 1960's,, I was baffled by the behavior of some of my classmates, such as being nonverbal, not talking, making loud noises, yelling, being aggressive, and not focusing or comprehending typical instructions.

As a kid, I didn't understand the behavior and the adults around me apparently didn't either. Interactions with the student with a different behavior pattern never transpired; the teachers would distribute school supplies to the students but not to those on the 'spectrum'.

The teacher did not have any training or support during that time frame. The majority of the students on the spectrum was left unattended and ignored. The other students would laugh and make fun of these students and call them disrespectful names.

As a peer, I also witnessed verbal abuse from the teachers, other students, and staff, and negative behaviors such as being afraid to sit near my classmate. Sometimes, the student became very aggressive, hitting, throwing, kicking, biting, and pulling another student's hair and not sharing any items.

There were also incidents when a student would repeat what our teacher instructed the class to complete. We, as students, would stare, make fun of the individuals, and laugh at our peers. We all thought that our peers would be having a temper tantrum as

Chapter 4: From An Outside Perspective

we described the behavior. The actual terminology is a *meltdown*.

As an adult, learning more about children with autism has helped me to become a better advocate for those students who do not have a voice to speak out for themselves. I guess you can say it was my own experience that changed my heart. I'll explain more later.

From my studies, I learned there are approximately 3 main symptoms of autism spectrum disorder, according to the National Institute of Mental Health:

1. Need help with communication and interacting with other people.

2. Restricted entrances and repetitive behavior.

3. Symptoms that affect their ability to function in school, work, and other areas of life.

Early detection and intervention, which I believe is what this book is all about, will help not only improve the lifestyle of the child on the spectrum, but also those of the caregivers.

DOES AUTISM RUN IN FAMILIES?

Yes, autism can run in families. Studies suggest that there is a genetic component to the disorder, so if you have a family history of autism, there may be a higher risk that your child could also have autism. However, many other factors can contribute to the risk of autism, so discussing any concerns and questions with your doctor is important.

An increasing number of people have received an autism diagnosis in recent years. It's fascinating that only a few years ago, autism did not appear to be as common in society. The cause of autism must be looked at to determine why it is more prevalent.

Although the precise cause of autism is unknown, genetics is currently the most likely idea. Understanding the causes of autism will advance studies into possible reasons why the number of people with the condition may be rising.

My Grandson (Kingston): When King was approximately 5 months old, he was not sitting up independently; we quickly realized that taking more time than normal would help the baby with his motor skills, such as prompting the bottle up and putting pillows up to assist.

Repeating exercises went on 6 months, 9 months, 12 months, etc. Once Kingston turned 2 years old, his speech improved; he began potty training, playing games, learning colors, counting numbers, using coloring books, and learning the alphabet. Using the correct English speech.

Kingston started Pre-K three years later, and he is doing phenomenon--writing his name; the alphabet is capital and lowercase, identifying all his colors and numbers, learning how to complete a full sentence, sounding out words, tying his shoe, bowling and being very competitive; he has mastered navigating through any phone or iPad.

From what I gathered as an educator who has been in education for more than 20 years, I have viewed autism from an outside perspective. Still, I firmly believe it takes a village to raise a child.

I have been blessed with educating children with autism spectrum disorder inside and outside the classroom. For instance, my student in the Language and Reading class in sixth grade was a high-functioning student who was competitive in Reading aloud and completing the assignments first.

This student would also multitask, doing his thing with his toys and coloring all at the same time. And as soon as I give any instructions, he focuses on the lesson plan and helps his peers.

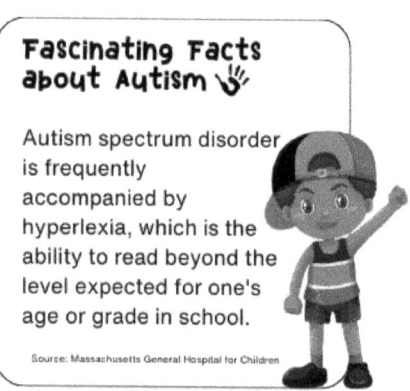

Fascinating Facts about Autism

Autism spectrum disorder is frequently accompanied by hyperlexia, which is the ability to read beyond the level expected for one's age or grade in school.

Source: Massachusetts General Hospital for Children

KNOW YOUR RIGHTS

As a parent and educator, knowing your rights, especially when it comes to the resources available to children on the spectrum is key. It can be the piece to the puzzle that makes life easier for both children and adults on the spectrum.

Chapter 4: From An Outside Perspective

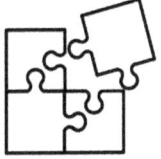

REFERENCES

Centers for Disease Control and Prevention. (2022, March 28). Signs and symptoms of autism spectrum disorders. Centers for Disease Control and Prevention. Retrieved January 28, 2023, from https://www.cdc.gov/ncbddd/autism/signs.html

What are the different types of autism spectrum disorder? – Onteenstoday.com. https://www.onteenstoday.com/samples/what-are-the-different-types-of-autism-spectrum-disorder/

Is autism genetic or hereditary? – Neighborshateus.com. https://neighborshateus.com/is-autism-genetic-or-hereditary/

ABOUT THE AUTHOR

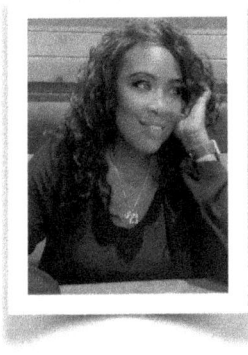

Evelyn Prewitt's story begins in Newton, Georgia, where she was born. At the tender age of two, her family, led by her mother, moved to Newark, New Jersey. Completing high school marked the beginning of her dedicated pursuit towards her goal of helping others.

Evelyn advanced her education by earning an Associate Degree in Criminal Justice and a Bachelor's Degree in Public Administration, alongside engaging in theological studies.

Evelyn's personal life is as fulfilling as her professional endeavors. She is married to a honorably retired Army Veteran, with whom she shares over four decades of military affiliation through her work. As a mother of two adult children and a grandmother, Evelyn finds daily inspiration in her family.

Professionally, Evelyn currently serves as a Site Coordinator for Communities In Schools at a local high school. In this role, she mentors students and promotes academic readiness, preparing them for college under the auspices of the Region 12 and Upward Bound program.

Prior to this, Evelyn dedicated over 20 years to the Killeen Independent School District, a tenure that heightened her awareness of community needs, especially mental health issues and the importance of belonging. This insight propelled her to become a foster parent, providing care to over 150 children for more than a decade.

Beyond her career in education, Evelyn is an entrepreneur, a minister, and an evangelist. Her life's mission is to uplift others through teaching, preaching, and embracing the word of God. She stands as an advocate for those lacking knowledge or resources to protect themselves.

Evelyn extends her heartfelt gratitude to her mentors and supporters: Dellah Fernandez, Rosa Velazquez, Mr. and Mrs. Burvato, Athenia Dorman, her daughter Ciani Pennington, and granddaughter Daejah Hackney, for their unwavering support and inspiration on her journey.

Conclusion

As we come to the end of this journey through the pages of "Voices United: Collective Excellence in Autism," we hope you've discovered the power of unity, resilience, and the human spirit.

The stories shared by mothers, clinicians, siblings, educators, and resource professionals have illuminated the path toward understanding and embracing autism.

In these pages, we've witnessed the challenges and triumphs, the heartaches and joys that come with raising and supporting children with autism. We've seen how rejection can turn into acceptance, how loss can transform into love, and how what may seem like hopeless situations can indeed be filled with hope.

But most importantly, we've learned that every child with autism is a beacon of excellence in their own unique way. Their differences are not deficits, but rather the building blocks of a more compassionate and inclusive world. As you close this book, we encourage you to carry forward the lessons of empathy, understanding, and acceptance. Let the voices united within these pages inspire you to be an advocate, a supporter, and a friend to those in the autism community. Together, we can continue to celebrate the differences that make each of us exceptional.

Thank you for joining us on this remarkable journey. Your support and compassion are essential in building a brighter future for children with autism and their families.

With heartfelt gratitude,

Voices United Authors

www.ingramcontent.com/pod-product-compliance
Lightning Source LLC
Chambersburg PA
CBHW041925090426
42743CB00020B/3442